REST, REFOCUS, RECHARGE

REST, REFOCUS, RECHARGE

A GUIDE FOR OPTIMIZING YOUR LIFE

GREG WELLS, PH.D.

Collins

Published by HarperCollins Publishers Ltd

First edition

HarperCollins books may be purchased for educational, business,
or sales promotional use through our Special Markets Department.

HarperCollins Publishers Ltd
Bay Adelaide Centre, East Tower
22 Adelaide Street West, 41st Floor
Toronto, Ontario, Canada
M5H 4E3

www.harpercollins.ca

Library and Archives Canada Cataloguing in Publication
information is available upon request.

ISBN 978-1-4434-5845-0

Printed and bound in the United States
LSC/C 9 8 7 6 5 4 3 2 1

For Judith, Ingrid, and Adam

CONTENTS

REST,
REFOCUS,
RECHARGE

INTRODUCTION:
GIVE YOURSELF A CHANCE
(AND THE TIME)

"This idea that unless you are suffering, grinding, working every hour of every day, you're not working hard enough ... this is one of the most toxic, dangerous things in tech right now. It has deleterious effects not just on your business but on your well-being."
—ALEXIS OHANIAN

Over 50 years ago, Sir Paul McCartney woke up and headed straight to the piano to play a melody that came to him in a dream. He didn't have lyrics yet, so he sang "Scrambled eggs, oh baby how I love your legs" while he tried out the chords. For months while John Lennon and McCartney attempted to write the lyrics, they jokingly called it "Scrambled Eggs." It wasn't until much later when Paul was on vacation that he wrote the words to one of the world's most beloved songs—"Yesterday."

Of course, not all breakthroughs are as big as McCartney's. Everyday epiphanies can be just as important. I was reminded of this recently when a young woman came up to me after a talk to ask for advice. She was struggling to concentrate at school. We talked about how the brain lights up during exercise, and I gave her a copy of my previous book *The Ripple Effect*. When she got home, she sat by a window with her cat and read the section about movement and learning. She then memorized a key section from the book in a single sitting—a skill that she had been struggling with before. The next day, excited about her learning break-through, she recited that key section of the book to her teacher and asked if she could use a wobble stool at her desk so she could move during class and focus better. The teacher agreed, the wobble stool helped, and her grades and confidence improved.

What I love about this anecdote is that it illustrates the power of simple changes in behaviour. Instead of being stressed or watching TV when she got home, she turned off all of her electronics and grabbed a book. She put herself in a relaxed position and engaged with nature through a window—and her performance improved. She had been struggling to focus in class—until she used a little movement to spark her learning. Little changes like these *can* have a big effect.

In today's hustle culture, it's easy to forget that inspiration and peak performance don't happen without helping your body do what it is designed to do. You need time to slow down, rest, and properly recover and recharge.

Even though we are living in the best time ever in human history, many people are struggling and feeling exhausted, anxious, and unhappy. We don't lead the healthy, high-performance lives we're capable of and deserve. We don't reach down to our depths and activate our hidden potential so we can climb to new heights. We're making five sacrifices:

1. We're sacrificing our health for our wealth.
2. We're sacrificing quality for quantity.
3. We're sacrificing response-ability for reaction.
4. We're sacrificing attention for distraction.
5. We're sacrificing internal motivation for external rewards.

The Path Forward

I see a clear way out of this, and it begins with our physiology. Looking at the fundamental changes that have been happening in the sports world over the last few decades really highlights how making simple changes to our habits can deliver great results.

When I was a competitive swimmer in my youth, and then coaching athletes in the 1980s and 90s, the standard philosophy was to train as much as possible: Lift the most weights, run the most miles, swim the most metres. I remember one training camp where I swam 10,000 metres in the morning and 12,000 metres in the afternoon . . . 4 days in a row. My events were 100 and 200 metres.

Back then, if athletes were lucky, they might get a massage at the end of a main competition or season. Stretching was optional, at best, and recovery practices consisted of some ice packs on aching joints. Often, the most successful athletes were the ones who were able to handle intense training without getting sick and injured. As a result, athletic careers were short, injuries were common, burnout was a given, and mental health suffered.

Fortunately, things have changed. We know so much more about human health and performance. Thanks to serious research into recovery and regeneration, scientists now understand that what athletes do when they are not training is as important as training itself. Think of NBA star Kawhi Leonard. During the season when he was with the Toronto Raptors, his sports scientist, Alex McKechnie, incorporated breaks into his schedule (now commonly referred to as "load management") to ensure that Kawhi properly recovered from his injuries, developed his fitness during the season, and then peaked for the playoffs—ultimately helping the Toronto Raptors win an NBA title. This idea of the "24-hour athlete" has become standard among athletes and coaches, who have learned about the importance of sleep, healthy nutrition, optimal training techniques, immunology, massage, and the use of heat and cold, among other techniques, from sports scientists. Stretching (now seen more as "mobility training") is used to build range of motion and to keep tissues healthy. Massage is a legitimate tool that can be used strategically to decrease inflammation. Cold-water immersion can activate the parasympathetic nervous system to help speed recovery.

Sports careers have become longer, and we now regularly see Olympians competing at the Games in their 30s and even 40s (and in equestrian athlete Ian Millar's case, in his 70s!). Where athletes used to peak once per year, many now compete at a high level on World Cup or X Games circuits throughout the year and then also peak at major events such as world championships or the Olympics. Perhaps most importantly, athletes and coaches are now working on optimizing physical, mental, and emotional health as a foundation for world-class sporting excellence.

We can break free from the sacrifices that keep us from reaching our potential—and it's the science and practice of recharging that will help us achieve it. It's time to take what we have learned from the sports world and apply it to our school, workplace, and home lives so we can get healthy, perform better, and ultimately focus on the things we really want.

It all starts by slowing down to speed up.

Rebuild to Recharge

I am a performance physiologist. My area of expertise is the science and physiology of peak performance. I love studying the human body and the ways different organ systems, including the brain, interact and shape each other for the better.

Consider your heart. It started beating about 21 days after you were conceived and won't stop until the very last moments of your life. During its lifetime, it alternates between relaxation (when your heart fills up with blood as it returns from your body) and powerful contractions (when your heart pumps blood to the lungs, where it is re-oxygenated and pushed back out to your body to replenish your cells). This relaxation/contraction cycle repeats over and over again—a perfect example of the balance between recovery and work. Upsetting this balance leads to severe illness.

Your lungs work in a similar way. As soon as you are born, you take your first breath of air, and you breathe continuously for the rest of your life. Breathing is a cycle where you contract the muscles between your ribs (your intercostal muscles) to lift your rib cage while your diaphragm muscle contracts and creates negative pressure that pulls fresh air into your lungs. Once your lungs are full of fresh air, oxygen is pulled into your blood and carbon dioxide flows from your blood into the air in your lungs. Your intercostal muscles and diaphragm then relax, and your rib cage drops and your diaphragm lifts, which pushes the carbon dioxide–filled air out of your body. The contraction/relaxation cycle then repeats. Upset this cycle and death quickly follows.

Your muscles are also complex machines that function best by cycling between relaxation and contractions. Your muscles break down adenosine triphosphate (ATP) molecules, which create energy to power muscle contractions that enable you to breathe, walk, run, jog, swim, lift, and play (and recover and regenerate). When your muscles rest, they clear waste products like lactic acid, carbon dioxide, and hydrogen ions so they can return to homeostasis (a stable, relatively constant internal environment). When we sleep, human growth hormone is released into our blood, which circulates to our muscles and stimulates them to use proteins to build new, stronger muscle fibres so we can exercise more often, more easily the next day. Moving and then resting and regenerating is how we get fit, strong, and fast. Skip the resting part and you minimize muscle growth and increase the risk of injury and illness.

The Power of Bioplasticity

The process where the body responds to a stimulus to repair and regenerate is called *bioplasticity*. You may have heard of a similar term called *neuroplasticity*, which is exactly the same principle applied to the cells that make up your brain (called *neurons*). Your brain repairs, restores, and regenerates both when you sleep and when you are in a calm, deeply restful state while awake. Just like the other organs in the body, the brain restores, repairs, rebuilds, and regenerates most effectively when we sleep and rest. When we spend all our time in hustle mode, cutting short on sleep, we end up with increased risk for cancer, cardiovascular disease, type 2 diabetes, and depression.

The really exciting news is that when we are stressed or severely challenged, and the body and brain are broken down, we can rebuild both to become healthier and stronger than they were before. This process is the key to growth. Think of this mind–body recovery and regeneration as a combination of neuroplasticity (brain) and bioplasticity (body) working then resting to spark growth. If we can consistently challenge ourselves and then recharge, we can activate bioplasticity and neuroplasticity to our advantage.

One of the best parts? These pauses to recharge don't need to be long to be powerful. For example, even a single deep breath can change your physiology and give you the time you need to compose yourself so you can respond instead of reacting. The positive benefits only increase when we deepen our efforts. Taking an unplugged vacation for even a few days can alter your mindset and open up your ability to learn and create. In this book, I'll show you why and how to build mini recharge moments (aka microbreaks) into your busy schedule so you can take control of your health, performance, and potential and create more magic moments in your life.

Slow Down to Speed Up

There really are simple, powerful, scientifically proven ways to improve and amplify your health and performance. In this book I aim to deliver both the science that makes it possible to achieve peak human performance and the strategies you can use to elevate your ability to reach your potential. Consider me your translator and guide. I'll show you the research, pluck out its most relevant parts, interpret it so it's clear and memorable, and convert it into easily achievable actions so you can begin to transform your life.

This book can be used as a manifesto and guide for helping you unleash your health, reach your potential, and experience extraordinary moments. While I do suggest you read the chapters in the order presented to develop your abilities to recharge, don't feel you strictly need to: Each chapter is self-contained and packed with information that will inspire you to action.

It is my hope that, by learning to apply the science of human health and performance, you will become sharper and more dialled-in, and will ascend to the top of your game no matter where you are or what you are doing. You will be able to maximize your performance in all key areas of well-being—sleep, nutrition, fitness, mindset, connection, and performance—giving you the strength, energy, and edge you need to achieve your dreams and goals.

Focus on micro-improvements. A 1% change may not seem like much, but each takes you, step by step, further along the path to optimal health and reaching your potential. I've included a series of 1% Tips throughout the book to help. Imagine how life would look 1 year from now if you had a 1% win each day for a year! Practise these tips and share them with your family, friends, and community.

Let's all slow down a bit so we can speed up.

STEP 1: RECOVER DELIBERATELY

"I absolutely believe that sleep is the most powerful, least expensive, most accessible performance enhancer you can get."
—ALEX HUTCHINSON

Why don't we have time to sleep? Too much to do. Why don't we meditate? No time. Why don't we go to the gym? Too busy. Meanwhile, according to the Nielsen Total Audience Report for 2019, the average North American spends more than 11 hours each day watching, reading, listening to, or otherwise interacting with technology and media, which is up from 9 hours and 32 minutes just 4 years ago. Simply watching TV takes up 4 hours and 46 minutes per day!

Imagine what you could do with all that extra time if you chose to do things a bit differently.

The perceived need to be and stay "busy" rather than spending time on important or fulfilling parts of life is destroying our ability to do our best work on the things that matter most to us, whether it's career, school, business, or passion projects. We are left stuck in our to-do lists and believing that there is no time for creativity, learning, exercise, hobbies, family, dreams, and, of course, rest and sleep.

Lack of rest and poor sleep then compound the cycle and it gets harder to regain health and well-being, let alone reach for more.

Sleep deprivation isn't pretty. According to the Centers for Disease Control (CDC), an estimated 50 to 70 million adults in the United States have chronic sleep and wakefulness disorders. Researchers at the CDC determined that among 74,571 adult respondents in 12 states, 35.3% of Americans reported having less than 7 hours of sleep on average during a 24-hour period, 37.9% reported unintentionally falling asleep during the day at least 1 day in the preceding 30 days, and 4.7% reported nodding off or falling asleep while driving in the preceding 30 days.

A study by Dr. Judith Ricci from the Albert Einstein College of Medicine showed that, over a 2-week period, 37.9% of the workers she interviewed reported being fatigued. Worse, 24.6% of the workers experienced associated health problems.

Busy people will often boast about how little they sleep. What they don't boast about is burnout. Scientists in Finland have determined that burnout and exhaustion increase the risk of mental and behavioural disorders as well as diseases of the circulatory, respiratory, digestive, and musculoskeletal systems. Burnout also has severe mental impacts and has been found to be associated with a decline in three main cognitive functions: executive functions, attention, and memory.

For some people, burnout comes from living a genuinely too hectic, overworked, and overfilled life—one that requires two parents to work full-time just to make ends meet while they raise their children, for example. For others, burnout is the result of adopting busyness as a value. Either way, there is light at the end of the tunnel.

A life of connection, purpose, and meaning cannot be built on a foundation of busyness. Rather, rest and recovery must be prioritized so we can achieve health and happiness.

PIVOT FROM BUSY TO DELIBERATE

In August 1954, a year and a half after he was inaugurated as the 34th president of the United States, Dwight D. Eisenhower visited the campus of Northwestern University in Evanston, Illinois, to address the Second Assembly of the World Council of Churches.

During his remarks, Eisenhower referred to a university president he knew who was fond of saying "I have two kinds of problems: the urgent and the important. The urgent are not important, and the important are never urgent." This phrase went on to become the basis for what is known as the Eisenhower Decision Principle—a decision-making process for prioritizing tasks and projects.

My take on the principle is this:

- Important activities have an outcome that leads to achieving your goals, whether professional or personal.

- Urgent activities demand immediate attention and are usually associated with achieving someone else's goals. Urgent activities demand attention because the consequences of not dealing with them are immediate.

I believe that Eisenhower's distinction can lead us to a fundamental shift in how we spend time that will improve the way we live, work, and run our organizations. We need to stop practising time management and start practising priority management. Moving from time management to priority management will help us directly address the burnout of busyness while indirectly improving the quality and length of our rest, recovery, and regeneration.

1% TIP: FOLLOW THE 1, 2, 3 RULE

To make rest and recovery happen in your life, follow my 1, 2, 3 rule:

1 hour: Spend 60 minutes every day on exercise, meditation, reading, journaling, or having a great meal with your family. Make a daily commitment to your recovery and regeneration.

2 days: Disconnect completely for one full weekend every month—no technology whatsoever. Read, go to the park, or ride your bike. You'll be amazed: Come Monday morning, no one will have noticed you were offline. Meanwhile, you'll feel a renewed sense of clarity and energy.

3 weeks: Take an extended holiday (3 weeks is ideal but take as many days in a row as you can). Collect your loved ones and go. Get off the grid. Disconnect. Go deep into a place of restoration.

DECIDE WHAT REALLY MATTERS

It's not easy to set daily priorities when you don't have a clear bigger picture. I can show you how much your brain and body require sleep and rest to perform at a high level. And I can illustrate how focusing on the important over the urgent will decrease busyness and increase meaningful productivity. But do you have a clear vision and a dream for yourself? All high performers do. What really matters to you?

Let me give you an example: Recently, I joined a group of scientists, doctors, and serious mountaineers who wanted to climb Mount Chimborazo in Ecuador. (If you take into account the equatorial bulge, Chimborazo is actually 2 kilometres higher than Everest.) It's a challenging climb: steep, dangerous in parts, and a very high altitude of over 6,000 metres at the peak.

The climb begins at the memorial site of those who have failed, and the psychology of starting from a graveyard is pretty bleak. Also, I developed some altitude sickness on the climb and experienced tunnel vision, dizziness, and confusion. There were some tough times. In the end, my colleagues Sara Thompson and Gillian White reached the summit while the rest of the team stopped just below. Each person on the expedition reached their individual limit at some point during the climb.

We were all able to participate in that expedition because of our clear vision: We wanted to be the humans closest to the stars (those up on the International Space Station don't count!). We focused on that during extensive training and the climb. That clarity kept us motivated. It got us up and it got us back.

Over time, exercising clarity appears to change a structure in the brain called the *inferior frontal cortex*, which is involved in attention control and decision-making. The more you focus, the stronger it gets—and so, of course, does your ability to allocate your attention to the most important things in your life.

1% TIP: REDUCE THE TIME YOU SPEND ON EMAIL

Our tendency to respond to emails as they come in leads to distraction and, ultimately, frustration over spending too much time on email and getting little accomplished. It is, for sure, not the best way to manage email (unless you're in the business of saving lives or dealing with time-sensitive material). For most of us, a same-day response is sufficient.

Bruce Bowser, founder and chair of AMJ Campbell, tells people that when he gets on an airplane he can bang out 30 or 40 emails very quickly because he's focused. There are no distractions. Go figure, right? When you're on an airplane, you're in an environment where you can be highly focused.

We can apply the same thinking during the workday. Pick the times of the day when you're going to respond to messages. You don't have to be overly rigid, but try to structure your time so you can be deeply focused instead of constantly distracted.

A lot of us get frustrated when our inbox fills up, either because we haven't given it the proper attention or because we spend too much time on email. Being deliberate about when you respond can alleviate stress and help you better manage your time and performance in the moment.

Consider J.K. Rowling, who was a single mother living in poverty and struggling with depression. Her first Harry Potter manuscript was rejected by 12 publishers, one of whom suggested she get a day job since she had little chance of making a living writing children's books. Her ability to persevere and remain faithful to her clear vision was key to her success.

Unlocking your potential begins with asking "What's my dream? What's my vision?" When you recognize what you need to do and how to do it, and can visualize the path forward, then you know what really matters to you. That knowledge gives you the chance to spend your time on activities that can move your life upward. In today's world of busyness, prioritizing recovery and regeneration is crucial.

As you adjust your priorities to add recovery strategies into your days, be sure to ask yourself what really matters to you. This will be the *why* that will drive your change and growth. When you know what you want and where you are headed, making the decision to take the time to recharge is a lot easier.

CHOOSE TO RECOVER DELIBERATELY

Managing our priorities effectively has the potential to radically alter the way we live. If we make conscious choices about how we allocate our time based on our goals and dreams—rather than those priorities imposed on us—we can improve our performance, relationships, leisure, and, most of all, our ability to achieve optimal health.

When we don't make deliberate choices about how to use our days, weeks, and years to achieve our greater purpose, we can end up like Alice in Wonderland in conversation with the Cheshire Cat:

> *"Would you tell me, please, which way I ought to go from here?" Alice went on.*
>
> *"That depends a good deal on where you want to get to," said the Cat.*
>
> *"I don't much care where," said Alice.*
>
> *"Then it doesn't matter which way you go," said the Cat.*

If you don't care where you're going, then there's no need to prioritize the important over the urgent. There's also no need to take rest and recovery seriously. But if you are working toward a dream, focusing on your goals every day and adopting mental recovery habits that support them is going to help you get there.

1% TIP: SET DAILY PRIORITIES

Managing your time is about fitting in whatever comes your way as best as possible. Managing your priorities is about deciding what matters most and allocating time to those tasks.

Beth Ford, CEO of Land O'Lakes, was quoted in *Fast Company* magazine as saying "I have a list of priorities that I make for myself. Every day when I get to the office I write down the top three or four things that I have to really focus on. This way I know what I want to achieve that day."

Once you have a sense of your goals—whether personal, professional, or organizational—you can determine how to get from where you are now to where you want to be.

We also have to remember to allow the process to happen and not look for shortcuts. Sometimes it is the process that creates the growth. When I interviewed Alex Hutchinson for my podcast (*The Dr. Greg Wells Podcast*), he mentioned that sometimes we just have to do the work and allow the body to go through its own natural processes to recover. Once again this means that we have to give ourselves time to rest and regenerate. We don't always have to get a massage. We don't always have to wear the compression gear. Sometimes it's okay to allow the body to get broken down and inflamed, because that's actually the process the body needs to heal and become stronger. It just takes time. If we're constantly cutting out the inflammation that happens when we train, then we don't get all the benefits of the training that we would if we simply allowed the body to recover naturally.

Being deliberate about how you recover, regenerate, and get healthy can make all the difference. Putting effort and time into the process is more important than worrying about the outcome, because process ultimately determines the outcome. Optimize the process and you guarantee the outcome.

REST, RECOVERY, AND DELTA BRAINWAVES

Sleep is when we recoup our energy levels and when our nervous system (the brain, spinal cord, and nerves that connect the spinal cord to muscles and organs) recovers and regenerates. When we rest and sleep, our brain activity decreases and electrical activity patterns slow right down. The activity that happens in a sleeping brain has been measured, with the electricity passing between neurons (brain cells) happening at a rate of 1 to 3 cycles per second (Hz). These are called *delta brainwaves*—the slowest of the brainwave frequencies (see page 19).

WORDS OF WISDOM: JUDITH HUMPHREY ON PRIORITIZING HEALTH AND FITNESS

Judith Humphrey is the founder of the Humphrey Group and a communications and leadership expert who has become an acclaimed speaker, author, and columnist.

It has been amazing. I am a different person because I've had time to commit to a healthier life. It's had a huge impact on my energy and sense of self. I now feel that I have this incredible perspective on what it means to be healthy and what it means to be truly alive. Even just the fact that I can go through a whole day without getting tired is such a wonderful experience. When I was running the business, I was always tired. I have found a new self from living a healthy life.

There is this wonderful energy you get from fitness, from exercise, from good nutrition. A wonderful energy that is a kind of life force. I really believe it can actually enable you to be better at anything you're doing in your career. I never saw that before. It's not just that you feel better physically. You feel better mentally.

I would say that if earlier in my career I had somehow had the health-transforming experience I'm now going through, I would have figured out how to make space for fitness in my life. I would have figured out how to delegate a bit more and let others do some of the things I thought I had to do myself.

While we are in deep sleep at night, in the delta state, our body releases anabolic hormones, which repair tissues and stabilize our energy levels. New connections between neurons in the brain are established and brand-new neurons are grown, which is one way that we encode learning and memories.

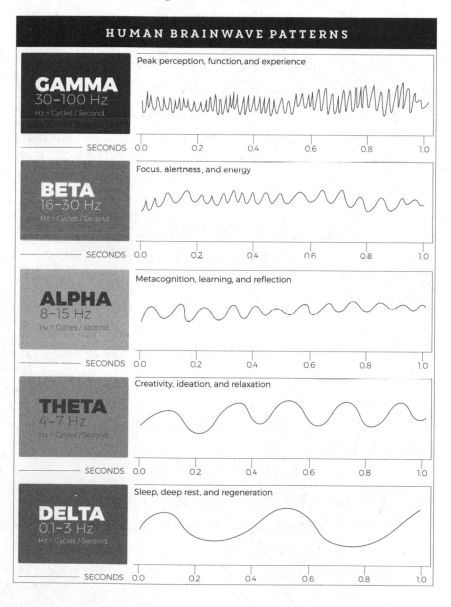

HUMAN BRAINWAVE PATTERNS

GAMMA
30–100 Hz
Hz = Cycles / Second

Peak perception, function, and experience

SECONDS   0.0   0.2   0.4   0.6   0.8   1.0

BETA
16–30 Hz
Hz = Cycles / Second

Focus, alertness, and energy

SECONDS   0.0   0.2   0.4   0.6   0.8   1.0

ALPHA
8–15 Hz
Hz = Cycles / Second

Metacognition, learning, and reflection

SECONDS   0.0   0.2   0.4   0.6   0.8   1.0

THETA
4–7 Hz
Hz = Cycles / Second

Creativity, ideation, and relaxation

SECONDS   0.0   0.2   0.4   0.6   0.8   1.0

DELTA
0.1–3 Hz
Hz = Cycles / Second

Sleep, deep rest, and regeneration

SECONDS   0.0   0.2   0.4   0.6   0.8   1.0

When we rest while awake—like when we meditate or pause to gaze out the window—the body and the brain take advantage of the decrease in activity to refuel and reset. We shift toward a delta state. Pausing to rest during our waking hours gives our bodies and brains the break they need to recharge and sets the stage for getting back into the higher activity states that we use to get things done.

When we prioritize rest and sleep and deliberately recover, we set the stage for better health and performance, and increase the possibility of reaching our dreams each day. It may seem counter-intuitive, but adding recovery to your day actually boosts brain-power, energy, and achievement. It's not time and productivity lost. It's performance gained.

THE KEYS TO REST AND REGENERATION

By taking the time to prioritize rest and recovery, you can unleash your potential to live a fantastic life. When you rest, sleep better, and allow your body and brain to recharge, you can dramatically improve your physical, mental, and emotional health, all of which set the stage for you to do what you love at a higher level.

To help you on your way, here are four keys to rest and recovery.

Key #1 (Brain): Recover with Your Eyes Closed

For most of history, humans have woken up and gone to sleep based on the sun's cycle. But our current situation is much different. Many of us work indoors, exposed to bright lights for 8 or more hours a day. In the evenings, we bathe in the bright lights of TV, computer, tablet, or mobile phone screens.

Our internal physiology is no longer matched to the rhythm of the sun. As a result, we're not sleeping enough and our health and performance are suffering. According to the U.S. Department of Health and Human Services, 20% of Americans have a diagnosed sleep disorder; 1 in 10 people suffer from chronic insomnia; and 97% of teenagers get less than the recommended amount of sleep each night. That's bad.

Along with sleeplessness comes increased rates of obesity, heart attack, stroke, cancer, depression, and anxiety. Lack of good sleep is so damaging that it actually shortens your life. An epidemiological study of over 1 million people, performed by Diego Mazzotti at the Universidade Federale de Sao Paulo in Brazil, reported that sleeping less than 6 hours a night was associated with increased mortality.

Here are just a few facts about chronic sleep deprivation, which the Centers for Disease Control defines as 6 or fewer hours per night:

1. We have higher levels of three inflammatory markers, including C-reactive protein, which is associated with a number of diseases such as heart disease and stroke.
2. For women, the risk of a fatal heart attack increases by 45%.
3. We have a 15% greater chance of developing or dying of a stroke.
4. Women are at a higher risk of developing breast cancer with more aggressive tumours.
5. Men have a 50% greater chance of developing colorectal adenomas, which are precancerous tumours in the colon.

Evidence also shows that lack of sleep increases inflammation and suppresses the immune system, which is why chronic fatigue is associated with heart disease, stroke, and cancer.

It's clear that poor sleep causes health problems, and sleeping soundly can help you live a healthy, disease-free life. But sleep also has a powerful effect on both mental and physical performance. This is true for exercise, sports, playing music, academics, business, and most other pursuits. Let's think about the positive effects of sleeping better and how that can help us perform better.

Many published studies have highlighted the importance of sleep for the brain. Dr. Hiraku Takeuchi and colleagues from the Institute of Development, Aging, and Cancer at Tohoku University in Sendai, Japan, performed brain imaging on 1,201 young adults and found that sleep duration was associated with greater density of neurons (simply put, more brain tissue) in the prefrontal cortex, where higher-level thinking occurs and dopaminergic systems of the brain (the parts of the brain related to pleasure and reward) are located. A negative correlation was found with sleep duration and density of neurons in the hippocampus, where learning and creation of memories are regulated. Basically, when we get more sleep, our higher-level thinking ability, mood, and learning all get better.

Philippe Mourrain, an associate professor of psychiatry and behavioural sciences at the Stanford Center for Sleep Science and Medicine, has suggested that the primary role of sleep is regulating the repair, regeneration, and optimization of the nervous system. He further states that sleep deprivation impairs performance on physical and mental tasks, while sleeping well strengthens our cognitive functions, memory creation, and ability to learn.

Professor Pierre Maquet from the University College of London has described the deep, slow-wave non-rapid eye movement (NREM) sleep that is more common earlier in the night as being crucial for encoding information and facts that we encountered during the day. NREM sleep seems to be when we establish new connections between neurons in the brain and grow new neurons in the brain, which is one of the ways that we encode memories and learn. The second half of the night—when we spend more time in rapid eye movement sleep (REM) sleep—is when we encode procedural memories like how to perform a new physical skill or mental process. It is also when we subconscious creative problem solving happens.

When I speak at schools I'm often asked about dreams. What are they? What do they do? The truth is that we are just starting to understand them better, and we know that dreams happen during REM sleep. Dr. Dierdre Barrett from the Department of Psychiatry at Harvard Medical School argues that REM sleep is "characterized by high activity in brain areas associated with imagery, so problems requiring vivid visualization are also more likely to get help from dreaming." We also know that dreams have helped people produce art, music, novels, films, mathematical proofs, architectural designs, telescopes, and other incredible inventions and works throughout history.

Scientists have discovered that Stage 1 of NREM sleep is related to mental flexibility (the ability to consider things from different perspectives) and creative thinking. Stage 4 of NREM sleep is related to originality. Another new discovery I found fascinating is that the natural cyclical pattern of sleep—the process of alternating between REM and NREM sleep stages during the night—is important for originality and divergent thinking (generating new ideas from many possible options), which is also a critical aspect of creativity.

You can make sure that you are taking advantage of these benefits by getting the recommended 7.5 hours of sleep every night. When your body gets to complete five 90-minute sleep cycles, your brain and performance will thank you!

Professor Jakke Tamminen at Royal Holloway University in the U.K. has performed some really interesting research on the link between sleep and learning. During Dr. Tamminen's research project, participants learned new vocabulary words. Afterward, some participants stayed awake all night while others had a normal sleep. Dr. Tamminen then compared the participants' memory of those words over two different periods of time: after 3 nights and then again after 1 week. The first-night sleepers remembered significantly more words than the participants who did not sleep on the first night of the experiment.

1% TIP: EXERCISE FOR BETTER SLEEP

A new meta-analysis (a study that pulls together previous studies in one topic, combines all the data, and summarizes the findings) has shown that exercise has beneficial effects on total sleep time, how long it takes to fall asleep, the quality of sleep, how much time we spend in deep sleep, and the quality of REM sleep. I have found that when I work out during the day, my time in deep sleep increases and the total amount of sleep that I need to feel recovered actually goes down (I wake up easily after about 7 hours of sleep instead of 8). Simply, if you want to sleep better, get some exercise during the day.

Professor Michael Scullin and colleagues at Baylor University in Texas did a different experiment. They gave undergraduate students with no previous exposure to economics a lecture on supply and demand. One group watched the lecture in the morning and wrote a test on the material in the evening. Another group watched in the evening and came back in the morning to take the test after sleeping that night. The test included some questions that were strictly recall and others that required integration of the material to solve new problems. On the recall questions, students who slept performed about 8% better than those who did not sleep between the lecture and the test. But more interestingly—and I think more importantly—students who slept performed 32% better on the integration questions where they needed to understand and then apply the information to solve new problems.

In today's world of smartphones, where the entire history of human knowledge is at our fingertips, the ability to understand and apply is more valuable than simple recall, and it looks like sleep can help us do that better. When you are under pressure, it can be tempting to claw back some hours in the day. But if you need to solve a problem or come up with a new creative approach, reducing your sleep hours is the opposite of what your brain and body need. The more you can commit to getting a proper amount of sleep, the healthier and more effective you will be.

In summary, a good night's sleep:

- reduces the risk factors associated with heart attacks, strokes, and cancer;
- strengthens your immune system, helping to keep colds, flu bugs, inflammation, and infection at bay;

- builds muscle via human growth hormone release;
- regulates appetite via regulation of leptin and ghrelin (our "hunger and satiety hormones");
- creates the conditions to help your brain regenerate via activation of the glymphatic system; and
- boosts learning, problem-solving, and creativity via neurogenesis and new neural connections.

It's time to prioritize sleep as the foundation for your health, performance, and human potential. And remember: Make 1% improvements. You can't do everything at once.

A simple bedtime protocol to help you sleep better
As the foundation of all health and performance, sleep is something you need to take seriously. And while you may not have access to a sleep coach like pro sports teams do, you can still put a protocol in place—a routine you repeat before you go to bed each night—to help you achieve optimal sleep so you can be your absolute best on a consistent basis. Here are four guidelines that you can use to craft your sleep routine.

1. **Work out during the day.** Sleep is enhanced by exercise. Any type of exercise improves the quality and quantity of your sleep. I have learned that when I do hard, intense workouts, I increase my deep sleep by about an hour compared to those days when I don't exercise or do light workouts.
2. **No caffeine after 2 p.m.** Imbibing caffeine in the morning and before important tasks during the day is fine for

many people, but its effects can last for up to 6 hours. If you're having trouble sleeping, limit your caffeine to the morning and decrease your caffeine intake to less than 200 milligrams of caffeine (2 cups of coffee) per day— which is hard to do when you're tired from not sleeping.

3. **Create a digital sunset in your home.** At my house, we have dimmer switches everywhere. With two young children, we start lowering all the lights in the house by 6 p.m. to help them wind down. You can do the same in your home. Start to lower the lights as you are moving toward bedtime. Blasting yourself with bright light in the morning is actually a good way to help you wake up and get going. At night, it's the opposite of what your brain needs.

4. **No devices for an hour before bed.** Tablets, smartphones, and computers emit blue light that hits your retina and is converted into electricity, which passes through the optic nerve into the pineal gland. The blue light that is released by screens is problematic in the evenings. By using your devices close to bedtime, you are actually telling the pineal gland it's morning. It will act as if the sun is up and inhibit the release of melatonin, the hormone that controls your sleep/wake cycles. E-readers that don't emit light are okay but not great. Real books and a small night light by your bed are best. Do not read *The New York Times* or an industry report. Read something that helps to create a barrier between your day and your sleep. You can also turn on the night shift feature on your iOS devices or use the f.lux app or an equivalent on Android to turn off the blue light later in the day.

With those four guidelines in mind, here's the sleep protocol I follow at home. This approach allows my family and me to love life, recover, regenerate, reconnect, and sleep deeply.

6 p.m.: We begin helping our kids wind down and move toward sleep: Screens are off, we have dinner, the kids take their baths, and we read with them. It's an hour that we always spend together as a family. Don't watch the news, check your email, or scroll through your social media feed. For 1 hour before you want to fall asleep, read a book, have a bath, meditate, make love to your partner. Disconnecting from devices will put your body in a relaxed state more conducive to sleep.

7 p.m.: The kids are in bed, and Judith, my wife, and I spend this hour together, relaxing or perhaps doing some yoga. With close to a hundred engagements a year that require me to travel, this time is critical to Judith and me remaining connected and in tune.

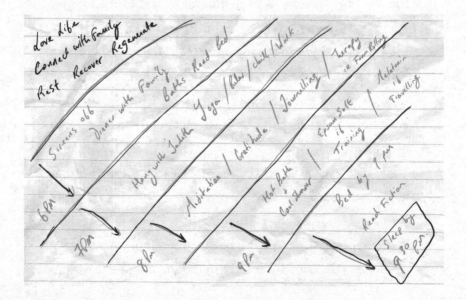

8 p.m.: Judith and I focus on taking care of ourselves (meditation, gratitude journaling, massage, or foam rolling) and cueing our bodies that it's time for sleep. If you are in bed and your mind is racing, making it hard to fall asleep or get back to sleep, try a relaxation technique like breath meditation, where you count backward and focus only on your breath. Reading fiction by a small night light, progressive relaxation, and visualization (for example, imagining yourself in your favourite vacation spot, in detail) have also been shown to help people calm down and fall asleep.

8:30 p.m.: To trigger the release of melatonin (the hormone that regulates wakefulness and sleep), we each have a warm bath for 10 minutes while doing a little meditation (see the Words of Wisdom by Dr. Ellen Choi on page 128), followed by a cold shower to decrease body temperature. (I also do this when I'm on the road and staying in a hotel.) This micro biohack helps ready your physiology for sleep without the use of exogenous drugs.

> ### 1% TIP: DEFEND YOUR LAST HOUR BEFORE SLEEP
>
> Many people struggle with waking up in the night. So many people wake up with their minds racing and then struggle to fall asleep again. If you are working late or thinking about problems in the hour before falling asleep, you will typically wake up because your mind is still processing that email you were trying to write or that spreadsheet you were trying to finish or that exam you were studying for. The best way to deal with this is to prevent it from happening in the first place: Defend your last hour

before sleep. Slow down and decompress for 1 hour before you want to fall asleep. If you do wake up, the best thing to do is to get up—*do not* look at your phone or tablet—and read some fiction or take a warm bath and meditate for a few minutes. Once you have relaxed, head back to bed to get a bit more rest.

9 p.m.: We get into bed and read fiction for 20 to 30 minutes. The body loves consistency when it comes to eating, exercise, work, and sleep. If you can adhere to a consistent bedtime, your body will learn when to release melatonin.

9:30 p.m.: Lights out. I wake up at 5 a.m. at the latest, so I get to bed early. After I wake up, I love to work out, meditate, write in my journal, and strategize about the day before my kids get up at 7 a.m. An early bedtime makes this possible.

No matter what you do, defend your last hour before sleep. Give yourself a chance to slow down. Allow your physiology to work the way that it's designed so you can get a world-class sleep and set yourself up to rock the day.

Key #2 (Body): Calm Your Nervous System

Stretching, building flexibility, and improving mobility are incredibly important elements of overall health that are often overlooked. Yes, there is an ongoing debate about exactly what kind of stretching is best, but there is little debate about the fact that we can benefit from adding some stretching and mobility practice to our lives.

The American College of Sports Medicine suggests that regular stretching can relieve muscle tension, reduce pain, and improve range of motion. In an era when activities like sitting compromise our health, stretching can be a huge help.

When done properly, stretching can also help activate your parasympathetic nervous system, which regulates recovery and regeneration. After a tough day at work, which I sometimes have, doing 20 minutes of stretching or yoga when I get home helps me to decompress and bring my mind back to the present moment, releases tension from my muscles, and begins the process of rest and recovery. The catch is that you need to understand what kind of stretching to do and when to do it.

Let's begin by looking closely at the two major types of stretching that have been the focus of research: dynamic activation and static stretching. *Dynamic activation* occurs when you extend your muscles while moving them to improve blood flow, range of motion, and potential power output (for example, doing slow but smooth walking lunges to increase your range of motion before a run). *Static stretching* is done while sitting or standing still, when you stretch a muscle and hold the position for a period of time (for example, touching your toes, which stretches your hamstrings, for 20 to 30 seconds, until your nervous system calms down and your muscles relax).

Each type of stretching has an opposite effect on the nervous system, with dynamic activation increasing the activity of the sympathetic (performance) nervous system and static stretching increasing the activity of the parasympathetic (rest and recover) nervous system. My approach? Engage in dynamic activation prior to a workout, and use static stretching after exercise or as a means to decrease tension and relax your muscles and nervous system.

For our purposes here, I'll focus on static stretching as a practice to help you rest and recover. Your body will benefit from some static stretching—stretches that relax your muscles and calm your nervous system. By performing static stretches for at least 20 seconds per stretch, you will contribute to your overall joint flexibility and reduce tension in your muscles. I also love gentle static stretching in the evenings as a way to help unwind at the end of the day.

There is a nuance to the practice of stretching that is important. Takayuki Inami and colleagues at the School of Exercise and Health Sciences, Edith Cowan University, in Australia looked at changes in the activity of the nervous system both during and after static stretching. They found that sympathetic nervous system activity, along with heart rate and blood pressure, increased during the actual stretch and that after the stretch the parasympathetic nervous system became more active and heart rate and blood pressure both dropped. This change to a more relaxed state lasted for more than 5 minutes after the stretching had finished. So enjoy the pause after the stretch is over—that's where the magic happens for recovery and regeneration.

Similar findings have been shown for people who practise yoga and Tai Chi. We are fortunate to live in an age when the ancient art of yoga has achieved international popularity and there is widespread access to yoga studios. Yoga is a practice that will help you develop mindfulness and get in tune with your body—habits that are of great benefit to all of us. From stress reduction to various forms of emotional release, the effects of yoga or Tai Chi will improve your mobility and health and help you live a vital and healthy life. Try a few different practices and see what works for you.

1% TIP: ACTIVATE BEFORE EXERCISE

My approach to integrating flexibility, mobility, and stretching into training is that you can engage in dynamic activation (any motion that extends your muscles while moving, like swinging your legs or arms or doing lunges) before a workout and use static stretching (when you hold a stretch for a period of time) after cool-down.

When you practise dynamic activation prior to a workout, your body is better prepared for the more intense exercise that is to follow. In part, this is because dynamic activation sends excitatory neuromuscular signals to your body, which improve muscular coordination and metabolic activity. This activation also increases range of motion, blood flow, and muscle temperature, all of which help with exercise.

Here is what I recommend before exercise: Begin by warming up for 5 to 10 minutes with light activity (at around 50% of your maximum heart rate) so your muscles have sufficient blood flow, oxygen, and temperature to benefit from activation. Then find a warm place to engage in some dynamic activation exercises like walking lunges, squats, and arm and leg swings. You can find a warm-up protocol on my website to get you started: **wellsperformance.com/dynamic-warmup**.

A simple mobility protocol to help you recover better

On my website I provide a stretching routine. Perform these classic stretches to relieve muscle tension and speed recovery. You should stretch the muscle until you feel a noticeable pull, but not to the point of pain. Hold each stretch for 30 to 60 seconds. As always, consult with your doctor or certified fitness professional before starting an exercise program or trying this protocol. You can check it out at **wellsperformance.com/stretching-routine**.

Key #3: Nurture Your Digestive System

Never before in the history of our planet have we had access to so much food. Despite this abundance, many people are not healthy. Many of the foods we eat, especially highly processed foods, are high in calories but very low in nutrients, which can leave us feeling depleted and hungry. Simply put, we are overfed and undernourished.

Poor nutrition leads to obesity, which is known to cause heart disease, type 2 diabetes, and certain types of cancer. Obesity is also a cause of depression (and vice versa). Additionally, obesity damages muscle tissue, which in turn causes exercise intolerance. If it is harder to exercise because your muscles are damaged, you'll become more physically inactive, leading to an increased risk of greater obesity. These relationships cause the vicious cycles that we find ourselves in and make it seem almost impossible to escape.

The good news is that while poor nutrition is associated with a number of chronic diseases, good nutrition can do the opposite. Good nutrition has been shown to help decrease the risk of getting chronic diseases such as obesity, certain types of cancers, Alzheimer's disease, and cardiovascular disease.

If you can overcome the confusion about what is actually good for you, which foods can improve your health, and how to eat to perform better, you can take action and create a diet that will propel you to new heights. The following seven strategies can help (I cover this in detail in my previous book *The Ripple Effect*).

1. **Hydrate.** Make drinking water part of your daily routine. Get a water bottle and keep it with you, and fill it up a few times every day. Water is just as important at work as it is in the gym. Stay hydrated and stay healthy.

2. **Eat mostly plants.** Eating fruits and vegetables will not only help prevent chronic illnesses but will also help you power up your immune system, which fights off viruses, bacteria, fungi, and other invaders.

3. **Consume more nutrients and fewer calories.** Remember this formula: Health = Nutrients over Calories consumed (H = N/C). Choose nutrient-dense foods as opposed to calorie-dense foods. For example, skip the muffins and bagels and choose lean, healthy proteins and vegetables (organic, if possible).

4. **Eat anti-inflammatory foods.** Poor nutrition causes chronic inflammation. Eating a large quantity and variety of fruits and vegetables can help optimize your anti-inflammatory and antioxidant status. Simply put: Eat the rainbow.

5. **Eat healthy fats.** To decrease your intake of unhealthy fat, reduce or eliminate saturated animal fats, trans fats, hydrogenated vegetable oils, and processed foods. Add healthy fats—nuts, seeds, avocados, olive oil, and coconut oil—to your diet.

6. **Eat healthy carbohydrates.** Eating a lot of simple carbohydrates like processed foods high in added sugars can lead to a depression of the immune system, kidney damage, atherosclerosis, oxidative stress, and increased risk of some cancers. Incorporate healthy

> ## 1% TIP: EAT HEALTHY SNACKS FOR OPTIMAL PERFORMANCE
>
> Provide yourself with healthy snack options that will stimulate optimal performance. Overnight oats are a great snack that you can prep in advance and take with you. My team member Dr. Melissa Piercell recommends adding the following to a Mason jar:
>
> $\frac{1}{3}$ cup rolled oats
> $\frac{1}{3}$ cup frozen blueberries
> $\frac{1}{3}$ cup coconut milk
> 2 tablespoons hemp hearts
> $\frac{1}{2}$ teaspoon ground cinnamon
> 1 tablespoon natural nut butter
> Coconut milk
>
> Combine all of the ingredients in a Mason jar. Cover with coconut milk, and stir well (the mixture should be wet). If needed, add more coconut milk to saturate. Shake and refrigerate overnight. Enjoy, no cooking required. Will keep in the refrigerator for up to 4 days.

carbohydrates—quinoa, whole grains, vegetables, fruits, legumes, nuts, and seeds—into your diet.

7. **Eat healthy protein.** The amino acid tyrosine is a building block for the neurotransmitters that wake you up and help you concentrate, focus, and problem-solve. Reach for protein-rich foods—meat, poultry, seafood, beans, tofu, and lentils—when you need to concentrate, problem-solve, or deal with stress.

Intermittent Fasting

Remember that habits form slowly through deliberate effort and 1% changes. No person can revolutionize their eating overnight. It's all about starting somewhere and then building on that momentum. And once you are eating well, it's easy to keep the habits going and include other ways to boost your health.

Interest in fasting has increased as people look to change the size of their meals (thereby controlling their energy intake) and how often they are eating (thereby controlling their time feeding and fasting). The objective of these strategies is often to help prevent or treat cardiovascular disease, diabetes, cancer, obesity, and dementia. The evidence for the benefits of intermittent fasting is compelling. Intermittent fasting (IF) is an eating strategy whereby you alternate a period of time when you are eating with a period of time when you are abstaining from eating any food. There are several variations:

- **Calorie-restricted eating:** This strategy involves decreasing total calories consumed per day by 15% to 40% and then maintaining the decrease over time—what many people refer to as "dieting." While this strategy works extremely well for decreasing body fat and has been shown to improve longevity in animal models, the data on humans is less supportive. Calorie-restricted eating has been shown to increase the incidence of disordered eating and anorexia.
- **Time-restricted feeding:** Also referred to as "intermittent fasting," this strategy involves limiting the intake of food to a 4- to 12-hour window per day. Typically,

most people in North America feast while they are awake (usually 16 to 17 hours) and fast while they are asleep (usually 7 to 8 hours or less).

- **Periodic fasting:** No or few calories are consumed for 1 to several days, followed by eating normally on the other days. For example, alternating 1 day of only 25% of usual intake with 1 day without restrictions. Studies on rodents indicate that periodic fasting may extend lifespan and protect against obesity, cardiovascular disease, hypertension, diabetes, and neurodegenerative diseases, as well as slow the growth of tumours. Human studies have been promising in terms of weight loss and cardiometabolic health, including reduction in body weight and improved lipid profiles, lower blood pressure, and increased insulin sensitivity, although implementing this strategy over the long term has proven challenging for people.

Anissa Cherif from the Athlete Health and Performance Research Center at Aspetar Qatar Orthopaedic and Sports Medicine Hospital in Doha, Qatar, conducted a fascinating study on time-restricted feeding (fasting) during Ramadan. Following tradition, participants didn't eat from sun up (dawn) to nightfall (sunset). After Ramadan, researchers found that participants had a 50% reduction in markers of inflammation in their bodies and that those markers persisted for months. It was as if the people who fasted had rested the inflammatory mechanisms inside their bodies! It's amazing how these ancient religious practices were rooted in a foundation for improving health.

A different study by Andrea Di Francesco and her colleagues at the National Institutes of Health in Baltimore, Maryland, showed that either reducing the amount of food we eat or changing the timing of our meals—adding a fasting cycle into our day—can delay the onset and progression of diseases and lead to a healthier, longer life. Positive effects on the body include decreased inflammation, oxidative stress, resting heart rate, blood pressure, and insulin production and increased cognitive function and stress resistance.

A related impact of time-restricted feeding is that it increases *autophagy*, which refers to how the body detects broken-down cells, breaks them up, and uses those pieces to recreate other parts of the body so the entire system can be healthy, strong, and fit for a long time. "Our findings show that the body has a built-in mechanism for cranking up the molecular machinery responsible for waste-protein removal that is so critical for the cells' ability to adapt to new conditions," said Alfred Goldberg, senior author on the study and professor of cell biology at the Blavatnik Institute at Harvard Medical School. Pairing time-restricted feeding with exercise appears to enhance this process in humans.

The combination of fasting and exercise also stimulates neurogenesis (the growth of new neurons inside the brain). It's really quite powerful, and the mechanisms through which that happens increase brain-derived neurotrophic factor (BDNF), which is linked to reducing depression and the prevention of Alzheimer's disease.

Think about how easily you can trigger these cascading positive outcomes: Simply eat all of the food you need (note "need" *not* "want") within a 4- to 12-hour window. Intermittent fasting does require a change in mindset and some planning ahead, but the only tweak you're really making here is timing. That's within your control and doable.

A simple intermittent fasting protocol to help you get healthier
If you want to take advantage of the benefits of fasting, you need to experiment and find a way to do it that works for you. Just explore ways to extend the period of time when you are not eating while still getting the nutrition you need to improve your health and performance.

For example, I often don't eat after 4 p.m. I am an "up early, eat early" kind of guy, so when I am fasting, I do it from late afternoon until morning. The other option is to skip breakfast and have your first meal at 10 a.m. I know a lot of people who prefer this option. Note that there is evidence that skipping breakfast as a fasting strategy does not yield the same gains when it comes to glucose regulation and weight loss as does skipping meals later in the day.

Research also indicates that to achieve greater physiological improvements, you need to go past the 12:12 ratio and get to a 16:8 ratio: 16 hours of fasting combined with eating inside an 8-hour window. If you really want to up-level this strategy, the research says you can add exercise. If you combine the 16:8 ratio with a workout, your body's physiology transforms.

When you give your digestive system an opportunity to rest, that cues the parasympathetic nervous system, which then drives your ability to rebuild, recover, and regenerate. Give it a try and see what works for you.

Please remember that fasting strategies are experimental in nature and should be done under medical supervision. Also note that children should not skip breakfast or fast. The research is absolutely clear: Children need to eat first thing in the morning or their academic performance suffers. My opinion is that no one under the age of 21 should be practising fasting unless they are doing so for medical reasons under the supervision of a physician.

Key #4 (Practice): Take a Real Vacation to Rest and Recover

When was the last time you took a truly relaxing, restorative, health-building vacation? I'm talking computer off and time completely away from normal life. Before you answer, check all of the points below that applied to your vacation time:

- ❏ You were entirely "unproductive." You may have been engaged in meaningful and even challenging activities (running a 10K, learning how to scuba dive, cooking French cuisine), but you did not contribute toward your work life.
- ❏ You didn't feel stressed or worry about what was happening in the "real world."
- ❏ You didn't check email or other work-related communications.
- ❏ You made arrangements in advance to arrive back to an empty email inbox.
- ❏ You returned home and to work feeling like a new you.

That's the ideal, and although very few of us manage to check all the boxes, we should be aiming for it. It's not just to take proper care of yourself and your loved ones—which is important—but also to improve your focus, work performance, and ability to pursue your dreams.

There is data to support these claims. Project: Time Off, an initiative of the U.S. Travel Association, reports that vacation use has been in a steady decline since 2000, from 20 days per year to 16 days per year, which is nearly a full week less than in 1976 to 2000. Recently, things have improved slightly. In 2017, 17.2 days of vacation were taken per employee, but a majority of the working population (52%) still reported having unused vacation days at the end of the year.

I'm guessing you're not surprised.

Our state of constant connectivity exacerbates the challenge of actually taking a break, and many people now consider the tethered vacation (that is, you are still connected to the office via your mobile device) to be the new normal. The thought of being "disconnected" makes most people anxious, so we either don't go away or we take our work with us. We fear we will return to a mountain of work, believe that no one else can do our job, or think that time off is harder with seniority. We want to show complete dedication to our work, and we feel we are expected to respond to work while on vacation anyway.

Aside from the costs to our health and happiness—and those are not small—the main problem with all this "can't get away" thinking is that it is founded on a myth. The myth is that working more makes you more successful and valuable to your company. But what if that isn't true?

Through its research, Project: Time Off has discovered that people who used fewer than 10 of their earned vacation days per year had a 34.6% chance of a raise or bonus, while those who used more than 10 vacation days had a 65.4% chance (for complete mind-blowing statistics on vacations, check out **ustravel.org/toolkit/ time-and-vacation-usage**). Moreover, an internal study conducted by Ernst & Young found that for each additional 10 hours of vacation time employees took, their year-end performance ratings improved by 8%.

A growing body of research is showing that strategic recharging, including all the topics covered in this book—sparking the brain with exercise, meditating to improve the ability to control your focus and attention, getting into nature to improve cognition—boosts mental and physical performance and, most importantly, health.

Changing work culture can also have a profound positive impact. In a *Harvard Business Review* article titled "Emailing While You're on Vacation Is a Quick Way to Ruin Company Culture," Katie Dennis offers two observations that ought to make business leaders rethink their go-go attitude to work: 69% of employees in companies that don't support unplugging do not feel valued, and 64% do not feel cared about as a person. These employees are also highly likely to be looking for another job. Trusting employees to handle the business while you're away provides them with opportunities to uncover new capacities and talents and develop skills, which grows your business.

In addition, as Srini Pillay points out in another *Harvard Business Review* article titled "Your Brain Can Only Take So Much Focus," being in work mode all the time exhausts the focus circuits in the brain, which drains mental energy and reduces self-control. *If you don't recharge, you can't use your brain power fully.*

Rest and vacation relieve our minds from constant hustle, which leads to better performance when we get back from the break. Recharging also increases creative problem-solving, accurate predictions of the future (better decision-making), and the ability to tune in to others (better collaboration and teamwork).

It's time to rethink the value of our vacations and start making recharge time a priority. Beyond taking proper care of yourself and your loved ones, there are so many good reasons to reach toward that ideal vacation I described on page 41. Research also shows that time away from work improves well-being, reduces the risk of metabolic syndrome, improves heart health, and might even be protective against depression. Although a shorter, less immersive vacation has been shown to improve health and well-being, and can even improve cardiovascular health parameters, the very limited amount of research done on this topic suggests that the benefits are short-lived (which means that as soon as you get home from your holiday you start planning the next one).

To fully recharge and activate your ability to focus deeply on what matters, you need to schedule many breaks throughout the year and/or achieve that ideal "away" state. Don't settle for random downtime here and there.

A simple protocol to help you take a real vacation
If you want to take advantage of the benefits of getting away from it all, you need to plan a bit and commit to actually taking a break. Communication is key in order for you to feel comfortable about being away and not needing to check in.

Here are a few ideas that can help you make a real vacation a reality:

- **Plan early.** There are good indications that the anticipation of a vacation is almost as important as actually being on vacation. Think about what you want to do, where you want to go, and who you want to be with, and share those ideas with those closest to you. Then start booking and scheduling.
- **Make sure your work will be taken care of while you are away.** Let your team, co-workers, and boss know that you are going away and won't be able to check your devices. Not every workplace will be ready for this, so do your best on this one. The main idea here is to build support for you to take that holiday. Just be prepared to repay the favour when your co-workers go away. Together, we can recharge!
- **Use your "out-of-office" email.** Turn on the vacation notice in your email, including a note that says something to the tune of "I'm going on vacation. I will delete all emails received during vacation, so if it's important, resend it to me on the day I return." When you get back, follow up on your words and delete everything. Start fresh. You'll be shocked how many people will respect your request and how few people will need follow-up when you get back—especially if you've set up the support while you're away.
- **Consciously disconnect.** Most adults don't ever make a conscious decision to disconnect. They are stuck

in a perpetual state of device addiction that becomes habitual, compulsive, and, ultimately, a drain on their resources and relationships. The hack I use to resolve techno-creep is to switch back and forth from being deliberately engaged to being intentionally disengaged. Decide when you are "all in" on the technology and get full value out of it. Then, block out time to disconnect, to be completely unplugged, at least once a day and in longer chunks over months and years.

That's it. Have a great holiday!

1% TIP: USE NATURE TO SPARK RECOVERY AND REGENERATION

Research clearly shows that being in natural settings improves health and reduces stress and stress-related symptoms. If you can go for a walk in a park or someplace you can see trees—or, even better, water—you'll reap the benefits.

THE TAKEAWAY ON REST AND REGENERATION

Sleep and rest come first in this book for a reason. The science is clear: Physical, mental, and emotional health begin with fully replenishing our energy stores. This too is clear: A life of excellence can't be attained without good health and the energy to live it. This is what I mean when I say that our physiology drives performance. Not just for athletes but for artists, executives, thought leaders, innovators, parents, romantic partners—all of us.

If you have a dream that feels out of reach, if you enjoy few if any exceptional experiences, if you are trapped in busyness, if you haven't ever or don't know how to achieve peak performance . . . I would guess, at a minimum, that you're just flat-out tired. Being tired sucks. It sucks the joy and potential right out of our lives.

Put simply: We don't have a chance to realize our potential unless we take sleep and rest seriously. We can only Kawhi Leonard ourselves to excellence by building load management, and specifically rest and recovery, into our lives. That means taking control of our physiology, our energy, and our environment and trading high stress, high volume, and high fatigue for high quality. Without rest and sleep, we can barely make it through a day, let alone change our lives, maximize our potential, and have exceptional experiences.

You may struggle to change your sleep and rest habits, but you *can* do it. You're in control. There are a lot of things we can't control in life—like when that hurricane blew through and ripped the roof off your house or when someone in your life gets sick. You know what I mean. But there's a lot we can control. It's within our power to build rest and recovery into our lives. It's within our power to optimize our own lives. Start now with sleep, rest, and recovery.

STEP 2: THINK ABOUT HOW YOU THINK

"Your unique power of reflectiveness—your ability to look at yourself, the world around you, and the relationship between you and the world—means that you can think deeply and weigh subtle things to come up with learning and wise choices."
—RAY DALIO

For many of us, life is stressful. Too stressful. There just doesn't seem to be any time to take pause to reflect on our experiences, let alone strategize how to move forward. But deliberately taking that time out can help us improve our mental and physical health, perform at a higher level, and, ultimately, alter the course of our lives. We *need* to take the time to slow down and reflect on our experiences so we can set ourselves up to appreciate life and learn new things. To use a driving analogy, we need to take our foot off the gas and press the brake more often.

Stress is a cascade of events within your mind *and* body. It can be positive, such as when you receive a compliment from a co-worker—this is known in the scientific literature as *eustress*, or good stress. Negative stress, such as when someone criticizes you, is known as *distress*. Believe it or not, both types of stress are essential for good health, but an excess of either can be dangerous. Too much positive stress can cause boredom and too much negative stress can cause burnout.

Unfortunately, we all know what stress feels like: You hit a patch of ice, your car starts sliding off the road, and then you recover control just before you hit the ditch. Within seconds, your heart feels like it's going to pound out of your chest. Your adrenal glands have just dumped hormones like epinephrine (also known as adrenaline) and cortisol into your blood. Adrenaline and cortisol increase the activity of various organs, like the heart and lungs and also your muscles. You feel like you're buzzing.

The benefit of hormones like adrenaline and cortisol is that they increase our capacity to function at a high level, both mentally and physically. This is a good thing in short bursts. But it's a bad thing to be flooded with those hormones for long periods. If they remain in our systems over time, or are dumped into our bloodstream day after day, they can cause problems. That's what chronic stress is—not just a short burst but a prolonged period of elevated stress.

That elevated stress over long periods of time—chronic stress—can make us sick. According to research published by Harvard Medical School, chronic stress contributes to high blood pressure, promotes the formation of artery-clogging deposits, and causes brain changes that contribute to anxiety, depression, and addiction. When epinephrine (adrenaline) damages your blood vessels, making them stiff, that elevated blood pressure increases your risk for heart attacks and strokes. And constant increased cortisol levels result in depleted energy and an increase in appetite, which can lead to weight gain and obesity. The American Psychological Association's 2010 Stress in America Survey found that 75% of people experience stress at levels that put them at risk for chronic illnesses including cardiovascular disease, type 2 diabetes, cancer, and depression. Chronic stress damages your body, threatens your mental health, puts strain on relationships, and takes the joy out of life.

When we perceive something as threatening, the brain will activate the body's immune system, which fights off invaders like viruses, bacteria, and other microbes. From an evolutionary perspective, a direct threat often meant that we would end up fighting or fleeing, both of which could result in an injury. If we're injured, those breaks, tears, and cuts expose our bodies to the risk of infection. The stress response evolved to keep us alive and healthy.

Inside our bodies, the sympathetic system activates our bone marrow and thymus to move white blood cells that fight infections into our blood. The lymph nodes and spleen, which filter our blood for invaders, are also activated. Hormones like adrenaline and cortisol further activate our white blood cells to make them stronger. Overall, it's like the body is preparing for battle, with all its defences mobilized and put on high alert. This is fantastic for surviving short-term threats, but we can't keep this system active all the time. If we're constantly stressed, our immune system gets depleted and we become susceptible to more illness and infection. Many types of cancer are kept in check by our immune system, so if it is weakened for extended periods of time, our risk of cancer increases dramatically.

When you are in a state of fight or flight, with stress hormones coursing through you, it's nearly impossible to settle into a state of reflection or increased awareness. Make sure you take some time each day to break the stress cycle and activate your parasympathetic system to rest. Doing this will allow you to cycle through periods of reflection throughout the day, which you need to understand all of the experiences and data you're taking in—in other words, to learn.

Let's explore how we can use stress to our advantage while opening our minds to reflection, awareness, and learning.

PIVOT FROM THREAT TO CHALLENGE

Research indicates that taking an active, problem-solving approach to life's challenges relieves stress and can transform it into something positive. If you withdraw, deny the problem, or spend all your time venting, you'll feel helpless. Instead, be determined to make a change, put effort into it, and plan for better results. Pivot from threat to challenge.

Our brains perceive a stressful situation as a threat. We respond to threats in our environment (a sabre-toothed tiger or someone competing with us for food) by increasing our ability to perform physically and mentally (run faster or fight better). We need heightened performance at times, but not all the time, which is often how we live—experiencing and reacting to various threats (demands, deadlines, presentations, running late, and so on) over and over again. Without time for reflection, we can't transform those experiences into meaning and learn from them. We can't change.

The daily and repeated threats we experience activate a cascade of events that involve the brain and body, all of which is known as the sympathetic nervous system response. The opposite response is relaxation and calm, which is regulated by the parasympathetic nervous system. Think of these two responses like the gas pedal and the brake on a car. The sympathetic system gives us bursts of energy so we can deal with the environment, and the parasympathetic system helps us rest and calm down after the danger has passed.

Being aware of the balance between your sympathetic (gas pedal) response and parasympathetic (brake) response is the key to managing your stress and being able to pivot from living in constant threat to taking control of your life and accepting challenges as learning experiences that move us forward.

Ultimately, taking control of our stress and our mental and physical states in moments of increased distress comes down to a pivot in thinking that allows us to view an event as a challenge rather than a threat.

When people experience a profound trauma, failure, or loss, they tend to launch into one of two trajectories: They either enter a growth phase or they fall into a negative trauma phase. One of the main factors in determining which direction they go is their perspective on failure. Those who believe that failure and trauma are terminal—incidents that can never be overcome—typically sink into loss and the belief that they cannot find a way out. Alternatively, those who genuinely see failure and trauma as setbacks, even when they are huge, typically enter into a growth phase. Those are the people who emerge from a crisis with renewed clarity about their priorities. They grow closer to friends and family.

They say, "I know who I am now. I have a new sense of purpose. I can focus on my dreams."

Practise Response-ability

Most people are perfectly capable of identifying the causes and effects of their stress. But what they often miss is that their stress is actually contained in their response rather than in the situation itself. Our stress is inside ourselves, not "out there." Negative stress occurs when you perceive a situation to be taxing or to exceed your resources. If you can shift your perception to see that situation as a challenge instead of a threat, you can make great strides toward ensuring a positive physical and mental response. By correctly locating your stress as generated internally, you can pivot from threat to challenge.

More often than not, the difference between a situation leading to eustress (experienced as beneficial) instead of distress (experienced as threatening) lies in how you perceive it. For example, anxiety is stressful but excitement is not; exertion is uncomfortable but freely chosen exercise is not.

Stephen R. Covey, author of *Seven Habits of Highly Effective People*, popularized an idea (likely originally authored by psychologist Rollo May) that challenges us to see that we can control our response to a situation. Rollo wrote, "Between stimulus and response there is a space. In that space is our power to choose our response. In our response lies our growth and our freedom." Sadhguru, an Indian mystic, echoes this concept. He suggests that responsibility can be reframed as *response-ability*.

This is a crucial point. So often we react to stimuli from our environment: Someone says something in a meeting and we react to that statement with words we might later regret. Or we react too quickly and with negative emotions during heated conversations with loved ones. We can also react to things we see on social media ("clickbait"). If we can pause for just a moment to consider what is happening to us, what we are hearing, and what we are seeing, we can respond to a situation deliberately and with intention rather than reacting with possibly inappropriate emotions and actions.

Imagine if we could build a practice of consideration before reaction. This could help us use our intelligence and experience to make ourselves better when we are under pressure. This simple practice of reflection, even for 0.5 seconds (ideally more), to create better response-ability could radically alter our interactions with life and the impact that we have while living. Response-ability is a choice; reaction is unconscious and therefore unreliable. Response-ability that leads to deliberate action can lead to excellence and profound positive impact and growth.

There will always be situations that seem like more than you can handle. But if you change how you deal with stressful events and shift from reactions to responses, you can begin to leverage the opportunities of challenges and the growth that can arise.

We are so locked in on the urgent things we think we have to do that we're missing the magic all around us. Spending some time on consideration and reflectiveness can lead to powerful insights about how we are living our lives or how we are working and what we could potentially do to make things better for ourselves, our colleagues, our loved ones, and our community. When we reflect on our problems and challenges in a deliberate way—journaling, for example—we can often put them into context and create maps to extricate ourselves from difficult circumstances or, even better, craft a new direction forward.

Leverage Radical Awareness

Some of my greatest experiences have occurred while travelling, specifically while out on safari in Africa. In October 2018 I had the chance to explore a national park in South Africa. Our guide led us through the bush to a watering hole, which is where animals come to drink and, therefore, where the predators and hunted congregate (ultimately, where the game of life or death plays out). We walked through the watering hole to the other side. As we climbed the bank and rounded a bundle of trees, I looked ahead and realized that we were 15 metres away from a massive, beautiful, and very dangerous rhinoceros.

In that moment, my focus was complete. I stood frozen, staring at it. I figured, "I'm going to die or not, but either way I'm getting a picture." So I snapped a photo and then we slowly backed away and moved to another area. It was so awesome to be in the presence of that magnificent animal.

When I got back to my room that night, I flipped through my pictures and looked at the shot of the rhino. I realized that there wasn't just one rhino in the picture—there were two. Not only that, but there was a beautiful green parrot in the frame. I had completely missed them. Sure, I was in survival mode, but because I was so locked in, I had completely missed what was happening around me.

Taking the time to be quiet and consider or plan something can trigger a reflective state, as can journaling or sitting down to deconstruct a finished task. Museums and art galleries can also

1% TIP: ACTIVATE YOUR AWARENESS TO GAIN PERSPECTIVE

Here are a few questions to ask yourself that may help you gain perspective on your particular circumstances:

- What is happening in your life right now that requires greater awareness?
- Where are you missing out on the periods of reflection required to pivot from threat to challenge and to transform knowledge and experiences into learning you can use?
- What do you need to understand more clearly?
- Are you living the life you ought to be living?
- Are you headed in the right direction? Focused on the right goals?
- Are you fixated on the "urgent" thing right in front of you instead of stepping back, slowing down, examining your thoughts and feelings, fully inhabiting your awareness of self, and seeing what you really *need* to see in order to keep learning and growing?

work wonders to change your thinking and bring some inspiration to your life. Reflective states are ideal for processing our experiences, thinking about ideas, or thinking about doing something, rather than the actual doing part. This is why they open us up to learning: Awareness of our thoughts allows us to understand and construct meaning out of all that's happening in our minds and around us. It helps us gain perspective.

Reflection can occur when we open our minds, increase our awareness, and leverage metacognition (thinking about how we think—more on that on page 61) to improve our ability to learn. This allows us to really know and understand what matters most to us in our lives.

WORDS OF WISDOM: KUNAL GUPTA ON
FINDING FOCUS

Kunal Gupta is the founder and CEO of Polar, a global technology company that is transforming the digital media publishing landscape and that works with close to 800 publishers around the world.

About 7 years ago I got to a point where I wasn't sleeping well, I had stomach cramps from stress, and I was feeling mentally very challenged. At one moment, I was like, "This is getting to be a lot, and I'm not sleeping." So I took email off my phone, and the next day I felt a lot better. In fact, I finally slept. That became my new normal. Then, a few years later, I started to practise mindfulness, which helped me deepen my conviction to use technology rather than be used by it. Now I have lots of practices for mindfulness, awareness, and being careful with technology.

Awareness cuts through everything. It's hard to be mean to someone with the awareness that you are being mean. It's hard to feel angry toward someone when you are aware there's anger happening. Awareness is an important ingredient to live by. Once we're aware, we know why we're doing things and it changes all of our actions and interactions.

To cultivate awareness, I meditate quite a bit. It's become fully ingrained in my lifestyle. It's like keeping your home tidy or taking out the kitchen trash before it gets smelly. I do it every day. Then, on a weekly basis, I do a longer meditation or a group meditation. That's like getting my place organized.

Then, monthly or quarterly, I go on retreats to give my space a deep scrub. I've been doing this now for almost 4 years, and I feel it's sustainable and has given me a very strong grounding.

Retreat is a really useful tool to cultivate awareness. I started with structured retreats—yoga retreats or meditation retreats. When someone else is looking after your stay and food and schedule, you can go deeper inside and really process your thoughts. Recently, my retreats have evolved to be more self-retreat. I basically take 3 to 4 days over a long weekend, once a month, and disconnect from every person in my life. It gives me space to really go deep inside.

I wrote a blog post recently titled "Why Some Experiences Should Not Be Shared." In it, I explained that I went skydiving a few years ago and didn't tell anybody. What I was exploring, and have since come to firmly believe, is that when we experience something, if we share it right away, we stop experiencing it. We experience other people's reaction to our experience versus the experience itself. We lose the connection to what we find meaningful in the experience. I advise people to go have experiences with friends, family, or alone and learn not to share them. You'll find even more meaning from them.

REFLECTING, DE-STRESSING, AND ALPHA BRAINWAVES

As part of my passion for travel and adventure, my family goes to Nicaragua to get some downtime and to disconnect from our daily lives. We surf and ride horses in the jungle and hike. One amazing day I was off by myself on a trail and I came to a beach that was surrounded by cliffs. There was one trail down to the beach, and I decided to go exploring. The trail was sketchy and had a steep gravel section that required 100% of my attention to get down. My brain was totally focused and firing on all cylinders, and I'm sure that if we had an EEG machine to measure my brainwaves, I would have been in beta, which is the alert and focused mental mode. I was in full-on focus execution mode to get down the trail and to the beach safely.

Then the coolest thing happened. When I got down to the sand and walked out onto the beach, I saw only one other person—a local who was line fishing off in the distance. We waved and then I sat down to take in the scene. The Pacific Ocean was spread out before me. There were cliffs all around. The waves were crashing on the rocks. I looked out over the incredible vista in front of me. It was beautiful and mesmerizing.

I stared off into the distance. I could sense my mind calming and noticed I was actively processing my environment; my mind was reflecting and contemplating. Then, as you do when you are alone on a beach for some time, I began to think about life. About my family. About my work and career. About my health and fitness. I was able to reflect and think very strategically about all aspects of my life.

I had shifted from a stress mindset (as I was climbing down the rocks through the trees) to a calm and reflective state (once I settled down on the beach). That place, situation, and scene helped me activate the alpha waves in my brain.

Alpha brainwaves (see page 19), which measure at 8 to 15 cycles per second (Hz), tend to come about during acts of reflection and metacognition, which is when we are aware of our own thoughts. This can happen when you are tuning into yourself, checking in on your views and feelings, thinking about your thinking, perhaps musing over an idea or event—or staring out at an amazing scene in nature.

The state of reflection is a crucial mindset for us to practise if we want to take control of our health, our performance, and our lives (see Key #1, below).

THE KEYS TO REFLECTING AND LEARNING

Learning to be reflective is an essential skill if you want to contemplate, gain insights, learn, and gain perspective on your life. If you can pause for a moment, change your mental state, and open your mind to greater awareness by reflecting on your experiences and strategizing how to move forward, you can alter the course of your life, perform at a higher level, and improve your mental and physical health all at the same time. With that greater perception, you set yourself up to continuously learn new things. But how do you do it? The answer lies in the following four key mechanisms that can help you make the shift.

Key #1 (Brain): Activate Metacognition and Strategic Thinking

Achieving optimal health and performance relies on establishing an ability to activate the metacognition pathways of your brain. We simply can't be in hustle/busy mode all the time. We need opportunities to reflect, which activates our brain for learning. If we can trigger metacognition (thinking about how we think), then we can be strategic about how we reflect and learn.

Metacognition is a fascinating process that was defined by John Flavell in 1979 as "the knowledge you have of your own cognitive processes (your thinking)." He further explained that metacognition includes your ability to control your thinking processes through strategies such as organizing, monitoring, and adapting. It also includes your ability to reflect and consider tasks that you have undertaken. This is the process that speeds learning and improves success when we apply it to tasks and projects.

Research at Stanford University has shown that metacognition helps students improve their grades. Dr. Patricia Chen, a postdoctoral research fellow who led the study, concluded that "blind effort alone, without directing that effort in an effective manner, doesn't always get you to where you want to go." Her work showed that when students were given a 15-minute questionnaire about what they expected would be on their exam, what grade they might get, what resources would be best used for preparation, and how they would use them, they outperformed students who just got reminders about the exam itself by 4% to 5%. This might not seem like much, but in a highly competitive world, 4% to 5% can be the difference between success and just coming close.

Dr. Chen's study was echoed by work at the University of Newcastle in Australia, which looked at how 1,390 Ph.D. students managed their learning. It found that those students who were "constructively engaged" outperformed their peers significantly. Of course, this seems reasonable: Students who are engaged do better. The challenge is to make this happen for ourselves more often. This study found that by focusing on the technical aspects of candidacy, such as what exactly is required to complete a Ph.D., how one accomplishes those tasks, and when those tasks need to be done, students could dramatically improve their learning outcomes. Thinking about their thinking improved their results. I believe this approach can help us with anything: sticking to budgets, getting better at sports, improving our fitness, or building a business.

While metacognition has become a very important strategy for improving learning in education, it still has not yet reached other disciplines like sports, music, drama, and business. Thinking carefully about our own abilities and what we need to do to improve allows us to strategize for personal growth. Science is backing this up, and researchers have recently identified regions of the brain that are activated when we practise metacognition. The rostral and dorsal aspects of the prefrontal cortex appear to be very important for accuracy of retrospective analysis of performance, or thinking about what you did on a task. The medial part of the prefrontal cortex is involved in your judgments of your performance. Basically, we are finding the regions in the brain that control metacognition and the ability to consider, judge, and strategize about performance.

You don't need to know specifically what part of the brain is working to take advantage of this practice, but I know that when people understand the science—in this case the anatomy of metacognition—it helps them trust in what they are doing and practise better.

The benefits of reflection and metacognition are powerful and can also elevate your ability to help others reach their potential.

One of the most dreaded experiences in families, schools, sports teams, and businesses is being micromanaged (telling someone exactly what to do and how to do it in great detail, and then doing it yourself to make sure your way is followed). Micromanagement kills creativity and learning, and creates frustration and boredom.

Ana Dutra at the Harvard Business School writes that when leaders pause and reflect—which is very hard to do in today's manic climate—they are better able to understand their role and empower others to be the best they can be at any task or project. She suggests that the pause-and-reflect process creates the space needed to become more effective and sets the stage for personal and professional growth in oneself and others.

A simple self-reflection protocol to help you activate metacognition
Activating your metacognition requires you to relax your body while keeping your mind engaged so you can explore the things you want to achieve.

The first step is relaxing your body: Sit comfortably, breathe deeply, and consciously relax the muscles throughout your body.

From there, research suggests that you can shift into metacognition by asking yourself three questions: what, why, and how. This allows us to think about how we think. To quote Dr. Patricia Chen from Stanford University once more: "Actively self-reflecting on the approaches that you are taking fosters a strategic stance that is really important in life. Strategic thinking distinguishes between people of comparable ability and effort. This can make the difference between people who achieve and people who have the potential to achieve, but don't."

Schedule in some time to pause and reflect: 15 minutes shortly after you wake up or arrive at school or work can be very helpful. When you are beginning a new task or project, take a few minutes to ask what, why, and how am I going to get this done? What exactly is involved in this task? Why is it happening—what is the larger plan or purpose? How will I proceed—what steps should I take? A what-why-how reflection helps to transform your potential into real achievement.

> ## 1% TIP: ACTIVATE METACOGNITION WITH THREE QUESTIONS
>
> Learning to be reflective is an essential skill for achieving the kind of perspective that can guide and fuel you. To achieve metacognition, relax your body and ask yourself three questions: what, why and how.

Key #2 (Body): Activate Your Mind-Body Connection

When you move your body, you activate different parts of your brain. Different kinds of movement can have powerful effects on our mental health, lowering both anxiety and depression and making us happier and more confident. As a bonus, exercise stimulates the growth of new neurons, which is the foundation of neuroplasticity (the brain's ability to change in response to learning and experience). So what kind of physical movement will both stimulate growth in your brain and allow you to achieve a reflective mental state?

Research indicates that mild to moderate physical activity seems to increase brainwave activity and shift blood away from the higher-level thinking centres of the brain such as the pre-frontal cortex. In a very interesting study by Professor Heiko Strüder's team at the Institute of Movement and Neurosciences, German Sport University, in Cologne, Germany, 12 runners were asked to perform four modes of exercise (treadmill, bicycle, arm crank, and isokinetic wrist flexions), each at 50% and 80% of their individual maximum capacity. At 50% intensity, there was an increase in brainwave activity in both the somatosensory (body sensing) areas and emotional areas of the brain.

Beyond putting our minds more at ease, rhythmic activities also create changes in the body.

Our bodies contain a protein kinase called mTOR (short for "mammalian target of rapamycin"). Here is how Matt Kaeberlein from the Department of Pathology at the University of Washington describes its role: "Broadly speaking, organisms are constantly faced with the challenge of interpreting their environment and making a decision between 'grow or do not grow.' mTOR is a major component of the network that makes this decision at the cellular level and, to some extent, the tissue and organismal level as well." That means that growth in the body—both positive and negative—as well as lack of growth are partly controlled by mTOR. Cells that grow too much or too fast can be a problem for our health, so inhibiting mTOR has several benefits, including reducing cancer tumours and extending a person's lifespan.

Interesting and powerful research tells us that we can block mTOR and extend lifespan simply by doing aerobic exercise, such as walking, jogging, cycling, or swimming. Beyond mTOR blocking, we also know that when we engage in aerobic exercise, we create something called *AMP kinase*, an enzyme in our bodies that has a massive positive impact on everything from muscles to bones to the brain.

Further, multiple studies have determined that aerobic training actually changes our DNA. At the end of every DNA strand, there is a little cap that looks like the plastic end of a shoelace. It's called a *telomere*, and it holds your DNA together and protects it from damage. This discovery won Dr. Elizabeth Blackburn the Nobel Prize for Physiology and Medicine in 2009. As we age, our telomeres shrink, and once they shrink enough, our DNA starts to fray and come apart, which causes errors to start to accumulate.

Telomeres can also be damaged by inflammation that accompanies being sedentary and eating highly processed foods, but by getting a bit of exercise we can often reverse the negative effects of not having previously gotten enough exercise. In recent studies, researchers compared the telomeres of runners (with an average age of 42) to more sedentary non-runners (with an average age of 39). They found that endurance exercise appeared to protect the telomeres in the DNA of the runners, even if they had started running at an older age. Physical activity can literally change your genetics at a foundational level. It's never too late to get started.

But you don't need to be a runner. Other activities have tremendous physiological benefits: Even a 15-minute walk can decrease your risk of cancer, cardiovascular disease, and mortality. And it does not seem to matter how fast you walk! Slow walkers experienced the same benefits as people who walked at a faster pace. Similar benefits are seen with cycling, so if you prefer riding your bike, go for it! Further, people who exercise daily have 75% fewer colds and flus—exercise facilitates the effective functioning of the lymphatic system in combating disease.

Another physiological benefit of physical activity is that exercise stimulates the release of stem cells, the incredible cells that can differentiate and change themselves into pretty much any other type of cell in the body. (My familiarity with stem cells is rooted in my time doing research with children who have leukemia at the Hospital for Sick Children in Toronto.) But stem cells aren't just an option in high-tech science. There's a simple way you can put them to work for you right now: exercise.

In adults, stem cells are stored on the surface of blood vessels in our muscles. Scientists have learned that when we exercise at a sufficient intensity to produce waste products like lactic acid (when our muscles burn) and carbon dioxide (when breathing hard enough to hear the breathing), we stimulate the release of stem cells from our muscles and blood vessels, which then circulate around the body and repair tissue.

Most forms of exercise have incredibly powerful life-extending effects. I encourage everyone to incorporate movement into their lives every day. It enables us to extend our lifespan, to enter a relaxed and creative state, and to improve our mind–body health.

Studies also show that positive changes in mood occur *after* physical exercise—and that movement is also associated with contentment and happiness. Recent findings published by Dr. Neal Lathia from the University of Cambridge in the U.K. have revealed that individuals who are more physically active tend to be happier in general. They also discovered that people are happier when physically active. In addition, it appears that an increased volume of physical activity is associated with higher levels of happiness. These findings were consistent across 15 European countries!

> **1% TIP: REFRAME HOW YOU THINK ABOUT EXERCISE**
>
> I have been exploring how a change in mindset can facilitate an improvement in physical and mental health and performance. It requires thinking about exercise in a new way: Instead of thinking of it as a "workout," think of it as "movement practice." For example, consider how you feel when you say to yourself "I'm going to work out" versus "I'm going to practise." The difference is subtle but important. I think that when you reframe your exercise sessions this way, you'll find that being active becomes much easier.

A simple movement protocol to enhance your mind–body connection
Physical activity calms the mind and decreases active thinking, enabling you to enter into a state of reflection and open up the potential for learning. Just about any activity performed at a comfortable pace before a mental task will enhance your ability to learn.

Researchers have proven time and again that exercise boosts learning. In one study, a research team divided students into three groups. The control group did nothing out of the ordinary; they just carried on with their schooling as usual. The second group walked up and down the halls for 20 minutes before math class. The third group walked up and down stairs for 40 minutes before math class. The results were staggering: Both groups of kids who exercised beforehand improved their learning and achievement—and the effect was dose-dependent. The more the kids exercised, the better they did at math. The control group didn't change.

Interestingly, the Athenians in ancient Greece already understood the mind–body connection. The whole point of their "gymnasia" was to prepare the body for learning. Students would come to learn and mix up their time in lectures and discussion with time spent doing gymnastics—stretching, jumping, bounding, and moving. Somewhere along the way, we forgot how to use our body to achieve a reflective state that makes learning from experience so much more effective.

Key #3 (Space): Leverage the Power of Nature

Significant scientific evidence supports the fact that spending time in nature helps us not only relax but also get healthier. Yes, forest bathing—and even river, lake, and ocean healing—improves mental health and human performance.

In a systematic review of current research (when researchers take a large number of studies and look for consistent findings across research groups and papers), it was found that immersion in nature improves mental, social, and physical outcomes. In areas with more green spaces, the risk of cardiovascular disease is decreased even after taking socioeconomic factors into account.

Research has shown that "green exercise" (exercise in nature) results in improvements in mental well-being, self-esteem, and even depression. This explains why trail running seems to help me decompress much better than running on a treadmill or even on city streets. Being exposed to plants decreases levels of the stress hormone cortisol, resting heart rate, and blood pressure.

One of the more interesting theories that explains the benefits of nature has been termed "restoration theory"—it highlights how simply viewing outdoor spaces has intrinsic benefits for our well-being. To stimulate deep contemplation and reflection, expose your brain to visual fractals—recurring patterns that are prevalent in the natural world: in water, trees, and mountains. Think of the beautiful patterns you can find in leaves, shells, and the starry sky. In nature you don't see the straight lines typical of an urban setting, specifically the consistent angles of modern architecture. This is one of the main reasons why practices like meditation or yoga are often done outside, in the natural world. Changing your visual field can trigger a reflective state.

What's amazing is that simply looking at pictures of nature can lower your blood pressure, stress, and mental fatigue—that's how powerful nature can be. So, if you're reading this at the office, change your desktop background to a nature scene, preferably one that includes water: Research has shown that images containing water are more restorative than those without.

Environmental psychologists Stephen and Rachel Kaplan from the University of Michigan have suggested that natural environments decrease stress and mental fatigue by promoting fascination, which allows our brains to rest and be more reflective. Think of the effect of closely watching a butterfly in a park or waves in an ocean.

Reflection and metacognition are enhanced and enabled by getting into nature, specifically lakes, oceans, forests, and mountains. A few years ago, near the end of an expedition to Ecuador, I went into the cloud forest up in the mountains. It's a rainforest that grows on the mountain at the highest elevations, where the clouds are. There are butterflies and hummingbirds, hundreds of plant species, and spiders. Standing there, I could literally feel my health improving right on the spot. Since then, the image of the cloud forest has stuck with me as a focal point for the health benefits of being in nature.

A simple nature immersion protocol to help you get healthier
When it comes to getting into nature, the research is pretty clear: More is better. But I realize that getting outside isn't always easy. Ideally, find 120 minutes per week to spend outside in a natural environment—that could be hiking, spending time in a park on the weekend with your family, cross-country or downhill skiing in the winter, any form of paddling on the water, going to the beach for the day if you are near a lake or ocean, or simply getting out of your workplace to spend a few minutes outside on a break.

1% TIP: LISTEN TO NATURE

Leave your earbuds in your pocket and head outside to the park, the woods, or the garden. Being in nature will lower your blood pressure, strengthen your immune system, reduce tension and depression, and boost your mood. To benefit from being in nature, you have to be attuned to it. Electronic devices distract you from your surroundings. To really boost your health and well-being, you need all of your senses soaking in the sights, sounds, smells, and textures of the earth, air, and sky.

If you can commit even more time a few times per year, leverage the "3-day effect" proposed by Professor David Strayer, a cognitive psychologist from the University of Utah who studies the effect of nature on brain function. Strayer suggests that 3 days in natural surroundings restores our brain function and sense of wellness. He hypothesizes that reflecting in nature allows the prefrontal cortex—a part of the brain where much of the higher-level thinking takes place—to calm down and rest. Camping is a great way to do this, or take a vacation by an ocean or lake.

Worried that you don't have time for 20-minute walks or 3-day treks that boost your health? Don't be. Research by Dr. Jo Barton and Professor Jules Pretty at the University of Essex found that the benefits of immersion in a natural setting begin to show after only 5 minutes. Sure, it's best to get out there for longer periods of time, but it's good to know that a simple walk in a park can positively influence your health. The greatest health changes happened in the young and the mentally ill, though all ages and social groups benefited. All natural environments were beneficial (including urban green spaces), although the presence of water generated greater effects. The authors call this "The Green Mind Theory" and are hoping that their results can be used to shape public policy and better environments where people live.

Key #4 (Practice): Eat Anti-Inflammatory Foods

One of the pathways common to all human disease, especially chronic diseases, is inflammation. Researchers have known for a while that inflammation is linked to physical diseases such as coronary artery disease, diabetes, and cancer. Scientists are also studying the role inflammation plays in mental-health challenges ranging from depression to schizophrenia, Alzheimer's, obsessive-compulsive disorder, and attention deficit hyperactivity disorder (ADHD). We also know that chronic stress is a primary contributor to elevated levels of inflammation in the human body. Given all of the evidence, it's clear to see that any conversation about optimal health and performance needs to include an exploration of how we can decrease systemic inflammation.

To give ourselves the best chance of avoiding conditions such as cardiovascular disease, cancer, and depression, we need to make an effort to effectively recover and regenerate. We can't unleash our potential if we're battling ill health, particularly those difficulties within our control. Each of us may have some physical or mental ailment that makes our lives challenging. That's the human condition—we have life circumstances to manage. But we don't need to pile on through false beliefs or bad habits. There is much that we can control and many ways we can optimize our lives. At the micro level, it's hard to build a habit of reflection and enter an alphawave state if we're tired, stressed, and unhealthy. At the macro level, it's even harder to achieve peak performance and exceptional experiences.

The science is highly compelling and clearly demonstrates that excess inflammation in our bodies is detrimental. The thing to understand is that inflammation isn't inherently a problem or even something we want to, or can, eliminate. In small amounts, inflammation helps the body heal, but chronic inflammation can lead to health problems.

Here's how the body's inflammatory mechanism works: Exercise and stress cause mechanical and metabolic stresses on the body, such as structural damage to cells and increased metabolic rate. The process affects mitochondria and produces reactive oxygen species, which are what we are trying to address when we take in antioxidants. Stresses also cause the body to release inflammatory markers (the white blood cells that go out and repair all the damage).

Ultimately, inflammation is a good process if your body can repair quickly. It's basically like burning down a forest and allowing it to regrow. You need inflammation. When you work out, you create inflammation inside your body. Then, through good nutrition and sleep, you cue recovery and regeneration so your body can heal itself and get stronger, fitter, and faster. But if you don't allow time for recovery and jump right into the next workout, you'll end up sick and injured.

The same goes for ongoing mental and emotional stresses. If you want to perform at a world-class level, you have to build in time to back off and calm down. It's really critical. A perpetual state of inflammation is not healthy.

Aside from adequate rest and good nutrition, there are lots of ways to reduce inflammation. For example, make sure your diet has ample vitamins, minerals, phytonutrients, and polyphenols (that is, eat lots of plants across the rainbow of colours and use many different herbs and spices), combine intermittent fasting with regular exercise (see page 39), and explore the benefits of heat (see page 134) and cold (see page 104).

1% TIP: LEVERAGE THE POWER
OF POSITIVE EMOTION

Anger, fear, resentment, regret, jealousy. When we let these emotions into our hearts and into our lives, they destroy our ability to perform. They instantly tear you out of the moment. Pursue a mental and emotional space of love, gratitude, and compassion, and you will achieve optimal health and performance.

A simple protocol to help you decrease systemic inflammation

You may be surprised to learn that what we eat affects how we feel—not just in the gut but in the brain, thereby affecting our overall mood and sense of well-being. Some foods are more likely to increase symptoms of anxiety and depression, for instance. If we're battling for our mental health, we're unlikely to be able to achieve the mind–body relaxation we need to feel deeply good and generate creative solutions.

Consider the field of nutritional psychiatry. Dr. Drew Ramsey, a professor of psychiatry at Columbia University, treats anxiety and depression in his patients with the help of nutrition. He believes that a poor diet is linked to depression—specifically, that the rise of rates of depression in the population correlates with the rise of a diet high in processed foods and low in micronutrients.

Here are some ideas to help you fuel your physiology through food, get healthier, and move closer to realizing your potential.

1. **Raise the nutrient content of your food.** I learned a simple formula for assessing the quality of food from Dr. Joel Fuhrman's book *Eat to Live*: Health = Nutrients over Calories. If you want to dramatically up-level your health, crank up the nutrient level in your food while optimizing your caloric intake. Then you can experiment and figure out how many nutrients and calories you need to feel great and get healthier. Look at your body composition and energy levels, and keep focused on getting as many nutrients as possible.

2. **Consume the right fats.** The science is clear that omega-3 fatty acids are amazing for your brain. My personal

experience also supports this finding. In 2017 I spent a chunk of time on retreat in Portugal, on an olive oil farm. We drank olive oil shots every night before dinner. I think I drank a gallon of olive oil that week. We would hike for hours each day and swim in the ocean. Then I would come back and spend 5 or 6 hours in their library, deconstructing everything I was doing with my career. I can't remember a time when I was so mentally alert and creative. It was amazing. Keep levels of saturated fat (fast foods, processed foods) on the low side. Instead, eat foods that contain omega-3 fatty acids (cold-water fish, oysters, wild salmon, shrimp, beans, nuts, seeds) and mono-unsaturated fat (olive oil, avocados, almonds, cashews).

3. **Shift from sauces to spices.** Move toward seasoning your food with spices like turmeric, ginger, and cinnamon whenever you can. They taste incredible and have enormous health benefits. Many spices have anti-inflammatory properties and loads of other benefits we're just learning about.

4. **Reduce simple sugars in your diet.** Sugar not only causes inflammation, it also decreases the size of the hippocampus, the structure in your brain responsible for learning and memory. Seriously scary. Just think about all those kids who are being fed high-sugar, highly processed foods every day. They're damaging the part of the brain associated with learning. I cannot believe we allow chocolate milk and pop in schools. High-sugar diets also decrease brain-derived neurotrophic factor (BDNF), which stimulates neurogenesis in the brain,

decrease cyclic AMP (the energy currency inside the neurons of your brain), and lower synaptic mRNA (the genetic code for neuron connections inside your brain). Sugar is bad.

5. **Avoid processed foods.** There are interesting studies on the link between an unhealthy diet and chronic inflammation in the body and brain. The most common dietary contributors to inflammation are refined carbohydrates (like white bread or pastries), fried foods (like french fries), sugar-sweetened beverages, red meat and processed meat (like hot dogs and sausages), and vegetable oils (like margarine). As Michael Pollan, author of *Food Rules*, says, "Eat [real] food, mostly plants, not too much."

6. **Eat anti-anxiety foods.** In an article for *Harvard Health*, Dr. Uma Naidoo makes a case for the important role diet plays in managing anxiety. She recommends foods rich in magnesium (spinach, Swiss chard, legumes, nuts, seeds), zinc (oysters, cashews, liver, beef, eggs), omega-3s (see pages 76–77), probiotics (sauerkraut, kefir, kombucha, kimchi), and B vitamins (avocados, almonds). All of these foods encourage the release of neurotransmitters like serotonin and dopamine, which improve mood. Foods high in antioxidants may also help: beans, fruits, berries, nuts, and vegetables like kale, spinach, and broccoli.

Try any combination of these techniques to decrease inflammation in your system, perform at your best, and improve your health at the same time.

THE TAKEAWAY ON THINKING ABOUT HOW YOU THINK

In the rare moments when I have some time to myself, I like to get up early while everyone else is still sleeping, make a coffee, and head to my backyard. There are very few things I love more than sitting by myself and watching the sun come up. This is my reflection and metacognition time.

The three questions of metacognition that spark contemplation and reflection—the what, why, and how—can make all the difference when charting a path forward in our lives.

We need time by ourselves to think, to consider, to plan, and to learn. In our hyperconnected society, alone time can be hard to come by, which is one of the reasons why we struggle with mental health. We are constantly in beta brainwave activity—hustling and racing around, taking care of our tasks and responsibilities. There is a time to be in beta, but our lack of alpha (reflection) time is killing us.

When we change our performance (beta brainwave) state to the thinking and learning (alpha brainwave) state, we can open ourselves up to a much higher level of performance and health.

STEP 3: PRACTISE RADICAL ATTENTION

"If we were to forgo our television addiction for just one year, the world would have over a trillion hours of cognitive surplus to commit to shared projects."
—Peter H. Diamandis

Do you know people with exceptional focus? People who have a mind-blowing ability to control their attention so they can stay with an issue or problem long enough to see solutions and possibilities that others can't? I call this rare quality *radical attention*—basically, deep and sustained concentration.

The ability to control your attention, concentrate, and focus deeply is a powerful tool for managing stress, directing your mind, taking care of yourself, accomplishing more of what is important, and reaching your dreams. It helps you to think clearly at work, at home, and while pursuing your passions.

In order to gain focus, you first have to protect your attention. You also need to be aware that we burn huge amounts of mental and physical energy when we are in deep focus mode, so it's easier to get tired and rundown—even sick. It's important to strategically recharge between bouts of focused execution (think exams, presentations, key meetings, workouts, etc.).

A great example of strategic recharging is el Bulli, a restaurant in Spain that was the subject of an incredible book called *A Day at el Bulli: An Insight into the Ideas, Methods and Creativity of Ferran Adrià* by Albert Adrià and Juli Soler. While it was open, the restaurant was widely considered the best in the world—2 million people requested reservations annually. Adrià, the chef, was known for carefully planning and preparing 35-plus-course meals. Through drawings, diagrams, research, chemistry experiments, even manufacturing their own tools, the team would be relentless in their preparations so they could consistently lead people through mind-blowing dining experiences. They ended up creating 1,846 unique dishes and became the best in the world at what they do. But get this: el Bulli was closed for 6 months a year. The most successful restaurant in the world was only open half the year. The team would spend the other half of the year deconstructing, planning, learning, and creating. That's a serious commitment to performance, recharging, and continuous growth.

We simply cannot hold our attention and focus completely on one thing all the time (unless you are a Zen monk who has been practising in a monastery for decades). We need to alternate between deep focus when we have tasks to do or experiences to enjoy and allowing our bodies, minds, and emotions to recharge so we can be ready for our next deep dive into all that life has to offer.

One of the most effective articulations I have seen of this principle is in a book titled *Peak Performance* by Brad Stulberg and Steve Magnus. They came up with a simple formula for performance that is incredibly powerful: *stress plus rest equals growth*. So often in the name of excellence we skip the rest and recharge part. We just can't. If you are seeking a life of peak performance and deep satisfaction, you need to hardwire opportunities to recharge into your life.

PIVOT FROM DISTRACTION TO FOCUS

About a year ago, my wife, Judith, and I were having dinner. During our conversation, she suddenly looked at me intently and said, "We need to talk." I slowly reached for my glass of wine and took a sip. Then she said, "I've got something to tell you. Something I have been hiding from you." I took another sip. She continued. "I've been saving $100 off every paycheque for the last 8 years. It's our 10th anniversary. I know you've always wanted to swim with sharks. I booked us a trip. We're going to fly to the Indian Ocean and swim with sharks."

Well, she certainly had my attention. I was really happy it was only swimming with sharks she wanted to talk about. But that was just the beginning.

We flew to a tiny island in the middle of the Indian Ocean, the huge body of water between Africa, Asia, and Australia. We arrived in the late afternoon. Shortly thereafter, Judith said, "Okay, we're going swimming with sharks now." We grabbed our gear and walked down toward the ocean. With the sun going down over the water, the island was perfect in every way. Dark green and blue ocean. Beach as far as we could see.

We met up with our scuba instructor and the three of us swam out into the ocean. I'm a swimmer, so for me being in water is like coming home. I was completely relaxed and just enjoying everything about the experience.

The current was strong, so we descended and held onto a wreck. I had a flashlight and a GoPro camera with me. I wanted to feel what it would be like to be in the ocean at night, so I switched off my flashlight. It was pitch black. I flicked my light back on, and we could see a mass of marine life swimming all around us. Turtles. Tuna. A clown fish swam right by my face.

But then I sensed something in the deep. I pointed my flashlight out into the ocean, and the light reflected off something shiny. I saw a tiny pinprick of light. I realized it was an eye. I moved the light sideways and it revealed a 6-foot blacktip reef shark. Harmless to humans, but it still captured all of my attention.

In that moment, I was ultra-focused, and I stayed that way for the rest of the dive. I will remember every single detail of that experience for the rest of my life.

If we can control our attention and direct it toward the things that matter most to us, we can experience life more deeply than if we try to race through our daily to-do lists. In this era of unrelenting distraction, attention is the one factor we can control that has a significant impact on our lives. Controlling and directing our attention is how we unlock our ability to truly experience life at the highest possible level in each and every moment.

What is happening (or not happening) in your life that needs complete focus? Answering this question is both a catalyst for health and performance improvements and an opportunity to break through whatever is currently limiting you.

Once you have the "what" clearly identified, you can develop the motivation to implement what I call the "focused execution pathway" to accomplish it by also identifying the "why." Successful people are motivated intrinsically (within the body and mind). They want to reach their potential because that's what they love doing. They are not motivated by anything outside themselves, such as money or the number of likes they get on social media.

According to both educational and sports psychology research, extrinsic motivation works well in the short term but not so well over time. Intrinsic motivation is a more powerful motivator for people over the long term. To understand your internal motivation, start by asking yourself *why*. Why do you want to eat better? Why is it important to prioritize sleep? Why do you want to get fit? Why do you want to improve your mental health? If you focus on what drives you from the inside, you will find it a lot easier to implement the new skills, knowledge, and techniques that you've learned to help you achieve your dreams.

Narrow Your Attention

States of deep focus often happen in the world of sports. Take, for example, the 2015 Major League Baseball postseason, during which the Toronto Blue Jays faced off against the Texas Rangers in the American League Division Series. At the end of the seventh inning of the fifth and deciding game, José Bautista came to the plate with the game tied 3–3, two outs, and runners on first and third. He proceeded to hit a 1–1 pitch deep into the left field grandstand—the infamous "bat flip" homerun. Later, writing in the *Player's Tribune*, Bautista described the moment: "On the walk to the plate, my adrenaline wasn't 10 out of 10, it was 10 million out of 10. It was so loud that it was quiet, and all that I could see was the pitcher. Everything else was out of focus."

For world-class performers in most disciplines, as pressure increases, attention narrows. In critical moments in your life, when you are under enormous pressure, you have to perform. So you narrow your attention.

In their book *Organize Your Life, Organize Your Mind*, Paul Hammerness, assistant professor of psychiatry at Harvard Medical School, and Margaret Moore, CEO of Wellcoaches Corporation, have proposed a three-step method to help prevent distractions from taking over your attention. They call it the ABC method:

- Be **Aware** (A) of what you are doing, what is going on around you, and what your options are.
- **Breathe** (B) and consider those options, even if only for a very short amount of time.
- **Choose** (C) thoughtfully: Where do I direct my attention?

When I was working as a physiologist for Canada's national golf team, the coaches and I would tell the athletes that whenever they got into trouble, they should ask themselves (and any referee that might be around) "What are my options?" When the athletes paused to consider that question and then acted deliberately, the outcomes were far more controllable.

Check out this extreme example of someone narrowing their attention while under incredible pressure: The first moon landing was fraught with challenges. Neil Armstrong and Buzz Aldrin, in the landing module, kept losing radio contact with the command module as they were descending toward the moon. The computer on the landing module kept spitting out an error code that no one had time to look up. To make matters worse, the area chosen for the landing was not flat, as the pictures had previously indicated; it was full of truck-size boulders that would have destroyed the lander. And they were running out of fuel. Through all of this, Armstrong fixated on a small field he saw where he thought they could land, and Aldrin called out data on fuel level, speed, and height. Despite the challenges and risk, they focused on what they could control, ignored the distractions, and stayed calm so they could perform despite the pressure of the situation.

The good news is that you can build your capacity to control your attention and strengthen your brain's anatomy, neural networks, and cognitive abilities. Professors Roderick Gilkey and Clint Kilts from the Emory University School of Medicine in Atlanta, Georgia, propose that you can improve your "cognitive fitness" by practising certain attitudes and lifestyle choices, and performing mental exercises like playing music, learning a second language, and taking dance lessons. Cognitive fitness expands our capacity to make decisions under pressure, solve problems, and perform to our potential even in stressful times. When we exercise our minds, anatomical changes occur in the brain that can be seen on an MRI!

Protect Your Attention

If you want to amplify your performance, identify what matters to you most and go after it with everything you have. Avoid spreading yourself around and letting your time and energy drain away. Decide what you want to accomplish and get on with it. Engage in single-tasking—allocate your attention to only one thing at a time—so you enter a state of hyperproductivity.

The same goes for your personal life. When you go to the park with your kids, leave your phone at home. If you want to take pictures, bring a camera and get your kids taking photos, too. The same goes for family gatherings like dinner. Don't bring devices near the table or even into the room. Put them out of sight so you can focus on each other and make that meal together special.

> ### 1% TIP: BE WHERE YOUR FEET ARE
>
> A popular way to think about living in the present is to "be where your feet are." I've heard this mantra from Oprah Winfrey. *Be where your feet are* simply means, whatever you are doing, wherever you are, make sure your head and heart are completely there as well—a mindset critical to achieving personal success and happiness.

By delineating times when technology is not in the mix, you get to purposefully decide when you want to soak yourself in it. Take an hour to connect with friends. Video chat with somebody you haven't spoken with in a while. Use your mobile device to learn. Find a cool article to read. Follow somebody on Instagram who inspires you. It's about intentionality. It's about connecting with life. It's about performing at your very best in whatever it is you care about the most.

Smartphones are one of the greatest-ever human inventions. We can connect to anyone, anywhere, anytime. Social media offers an unprecedented platform for the discourse, engagement, and awareness that gives social movements speed and force. Would #MeToo have been possible before the advent of hashtag culture?

Like many innovations, however, the ubiquitous and immediate nature of smartphone access has a downside. Our phone can pull us away from what is happening around us. We can end up at a magnificent concert and be more concerned about filming it than about taking in the performance. We can be perpetually distant from those around us.

Practise using your devices for intentional communication with the people you love. Intentionally engage with social media to celebrate and congratulate people on amazing things that are happening in their lives. If you cannot manage your devices with intentionality, you will continue to fall into a state of passive consumption, scrolling through your feeds mindlessly. When that happens, the behaviour is definitely controlling you rather than the other way around.

It's all about intention rather than compulsion. If you're intentionally engaging, you are in control, but if you are compulsively scrolling, you are likely on someone else's agenda.

Imagine how different your life would be if you ditched the mindless TV or news and instead watched documentaries or read biographies. You'd be in a very, very different place. This idea is called the *media psychology effect*. What you consume has a tremendous impact on your mindset and mental health. It's why I constantly encourage people to audit the media they consume and make choices that support their well-being and achievement.

There will always be a steady supply of every kind of messaging out there. If you want to consume hateful messages, they are there for you. If you want to participate in a culture where the game is to put other people down, you can do it all day long. Or you can decide that you will take in only what inspires you, puts you in a positive headspace, and gives you confidence and calm.

What are you listening to? What podcasts do you consume? What books are you reading? What are your kids tuned into online? Which friends do you engage with on social media? All of these choices influence your ability to surround yourself with positivity.

Take some time to go through all your apps, contacts, social media connections, podcasts, books, magazine subscriptions, and any other source of information or connection, and do a hard audit. Remove anything and everything that does not move you forward or could steal your focus.

Whatever it is you choose to consume, it's really important that it allows you to craft an amazing psychology for yourself through media and the people in your life.

WORDS OF WISDOM: JOHN FOLEY
ON HOW WHEN PRESSURE INCREASES,
FOCUS NARROWS

John Foley is the author of Fearless Success, *a Sloan Fellow at the Stanford School of Business, and a former lead solo pilot for the U.S. Navy's Blue Angels.*

Flying is a very calm environment. Not the first time, and not even the second, but after many repetitions, there is a point where you become very calm and everything slows down. I believe what is actually happening is the experience is not slowing down, your mind is speeding up. You're in a state of incredible flow and focus, where you can actually see the cracks on the paint of a plane flying right next to you at 500 miles per hour.

Let me give you an example of a performance situation. This is what happens in 16 seconds.

We've got 30 manoeuvres going on in the airshow. There's a diamond manoeuvre and a solo manoeuvre. Diamond means there's four pilots flying together in formation, and solos are two jets coming at each other to demonstrate maximum performance. We would alternate the different roles. When the diamond's in front of the crowd, myself and Thumper, my partner for the solo, are behind the crowd and getting set up for our manoeuvres. We're thinking about our preparation.

We've already scoped out the airfield weeks in advance. We've got photographs. They're much better now with GPS, but back then we would take satellite photos, and we would plot a centre point that would be a single point of focus. That point is on the airfield—it'd be a truck or tractor-trailer on the runway if we are over land or a boat if we are over water. We would draw flight lines and make tick marks—1-mile, 2-mile, 3-mile checkpoints. And there are 30-degree offsets. We map this thing out on paper—just on paper.

When I get to the show site, I have to be able to translate from a piece of paper to my mind. It's critical because I don't have time flying upside down at 400 knots, a hundred feet off the ground, to look at a piece of paper and go, "Hey! What was my two-mile checkpoint?" You've got to have that burned into your mind. On Thursday before the show, to prepare for flying at each other at 1,000 miles per hour, we would do the opposite—fly together over the checkpoint and hit the centre point. As we pass the centre point, we hit our stopwatch. We time for 9 seconds. We look down and go, "Where's our 1-mile checkpoint? Where's that road inter-section?" Then keep flying another 9 seconds and find the 2-mile checkpoint. And you put it in your brain. It burns into your brain.

I remember when I first joined the team and my mentor, Spurt was his call sign, comes up to me one day and says, "Hey, Gucci, as a 2-mile checkpoint, we'll use a white house." Now there were a ton of white houses out there. He said something I will never forget because it blew me away. He says, "We'll actually use the northeast corner of the three-story white house, the upper window with the green shade." I was like, "Are you kidding me? I'm flying at 400 knots and you expect me to see a green shade on a window on the northeast corner of this white house surrounded by a bunch of other white houses? No way."

But then I realized I was limiting belief. You can't do that—with the Angels or in life. It takes repetition, it takes practice, but I got to the point where it was natural for me to be upside down at 400 knots and pick out the green shade of a window on a white house. If you know what you are looking for and you are prepared, you can do it. Otherwise, it's a blur. It's the same in life: You have to choose what you focus on because it takes energy.

We do the preparation, and we are coming at each other. I have made a contract. I'll be on the flight line. Flight line is not the runway. Flight line is the inside edge of the left, painted stripe on the runway. My contract to my teammate is I won't be 5 feet left or 5 feet right. I'll be online.

I'd set the altitude and sometimes it's 80 feet off the ground. Then I'd give you a command, as you're coming at me, a command to execute a full-stick deflection rule. When I say "Ready, hit it," I don't care where you are in your life, you execute full-stick deflection rule, otherwise we've got a real problem. And I have to execute. *Bam!* We go by each other. It's a thump. As the airplane goes by, you have to rollout, you've got to pull 7 $\frac{1}{2}$ Gs, the Earth is coming down on you.

In 16 seconds, we have gone from 6 miles apart 'til we've crossed and cleared formation. I could break that down into fractions of seconds, 100ths of a second. I can see every frame in my mind and that's where it slows down. You're so focused that it's very calm. And you aren't thinking at all. If you are thinking, you are dead. But because you trained and focused, you can execute at the highest imaginable level.

RADICAL ATTENTION, FOCUSED EXECUTION, AND BETA BRAINWAVES

When we are in a state of deep focus and directed attention, neurons in our brain create beta brainwaves (see page 19), which move through the brain at 16 to 30 cycles per second (Hz). Focus and attention seem to be controlled by neurons in the superior frontal lobe of the brain, the inferior parietal lobe, and the superior temporal cortex. The inferior frontal cortex also appears to play a role in attention and inhibition (decision-making about where you direct your attention).

The goal here is to train yourself to control your attention and then recharge so you can continue to enter states of deep focus. Controlling your attention and energy enables you to experience life to the limits of your capability. Recharging your energy helps you to live life to your potential consistently, over time, without getting burned out and exhausted.

THE KEYS TO ACCESSING RADICAL ATTENTION

When you are actively engaged in a mental activity or task—having a conversation, making decisions, or solving problems—your brain is focused and attentive. Any time there is a high draw of mental energy—when you are making a presentation or a speech, teaching a class, providing a legal argument, engaging in debate, working with a group to solve a problem—your brain is energetic. These highly active states are great when we are performing tasks and getting things done. However, when we spend all of our time hustling, we inevitably end up feeling weary and fatigued.

The good news is that over time, exercising your clarity and focus appears to change structures in the brain called the *anterior cingulate cortex* and the *inferior frontal cortex*, which are involved in decision-making and the interpretation of information from the environment. When you practise focus repeatedly, those structures grow and strengthen—your brain actually changes. As a result, so does your ability to control your attention.

Key #1 (Brain): Use Mindfulness to Engage and Sharpen Focus

Few moments in sports can compete with the moment in baseball when an elite pitcher and clutch hitter square off during the playoffs with a game on the line. The pitcher's eyes focus on the target while they try to block out the crowd, the cameras, and the crushing idea that this is a career-defining moment. The hitter breathes deeply to stay calm and relaxed while trying to remain on edge so they can deliver explosive power and energy at that precise moment. Both athletes are entirely present. They are living purely in the moment, and that is a powerful learning point for the rest of us. In an era of constant distraction, the power to bring our attention into the present can be a game changer.

Mindfulness training is a powerful step on the path to increased focus. Mindfulness is an awareness of the world around you in the here and now, and it has two main components: 1) attention to the present and 2) acceptance and non-judgment. It's a practice whereby any time you notice your mind wandering, you bring it back to the task at hand and the current moment in time. Simply: "Be Here. Now." This approach was popularized by Jon Kabat-Zin, who was the lead in translating Buddhist mind training into secular contexts. He described mindfulness as "the awareness that emerges through paying attention on purpose, in the present moment, and non-judgementally to the unfolding of experience moment by moment."

There is no good or bad. You are practising living in the moment and controlling your attention.

There has been some confusion and overlap between mindfulness and meditation. Consider mindfulness as a practice of becoming aware of your mind, emotions, and behaviour, and mindfulness meditation (one of the many forms of meditation available to us) as a particular technique to help you improve your ability to control your attention and choose your mindset. Just as weight training is a program that helps to build strength so you can move heavy objects at will, mindfulness meditation builds the mental muscles required to attend to and adaptively interpret life's experiences.

The scientific interest in mindfulness has surged, which is great because it is helping the practice become more accepted in the West. The research has also now moved from simply show-ing the benefits of mindfulness and meditation to unravelling the physiological mechanisms that explain the benefits.

After 8 weeks of regular mindfulness meditation, the neurons and tissues inside the brain responsible for helping us stay focused grow and increase the number of connections they make with other neurons in the brain. In 2011, professor Sara Lazar and her team at Harvard University published data that showed how 8 weeks of mindfulness-based stress-reduction (MBSR) meditation resulted in an increase in the cortical thickness of the hippocampus (which modulates learning and memory) and a decrease in the volume of the amygdala (a structure in the brain that regulates fear, anxiety, and stress). These changes likely explain why mindfulness medi-tation improves outcomes for people with anxiety.

Mindfulness training has also been shown to be helpful for people struggling with addictions and eating disorders, attention deficit hyperactivity disorder (ADHD), recurrent depression, and severe mental illnesses, among many other conditions. Recently, the attitudinal qualities of mindfulness training were credited for driving many of the benefits related to increasing resilience.

Consistent meditation also appears to protect the grey matter in the brain from age-related decline. "We expected rather small and distinct effects located in some of the regions that had previ-ously been associated with meditating," said study author Florian Kurth, postdoctoral fellow at the UCLA Brain Mapping Center. "Instead, what we actually observed was a widespread effect of meditation that encompassed regions throughout the entire brain."

On the other end of the health spectrum, mindfulness is now becoming standard practice for progressive athletes and coaches to enhance human performance. Athletes are finding mindfulness and meditation training helpful for improving their ability to focus and control their attention; reducing anxiety, stress, and burnout; and enhancing their ability to enter into flow states. I have personally found it extremely helpful for improving my ability to stop negative self-talk that can happen during workouts and events.

The changes that practising mindfulness elicits in the brain—decreased activation of what is known as the "default mode network" and an increase in the activation of the "experiential network"—are quite amazing. You experience this when your mind wanders and then you realize you are daydreaming and bring your attention back into the here and now—that's the shift from the default mode network in your brain to the experiential network. With practice and consistency, other networks in the brain related to the ability to control focus and attention become more active and strengthened. These are the alerting, orienting, and executive control networks, all of which are critical for mental performance.

As Pressure Increases, Focus Narrows

Imagine that you are about to give a presentation to a large audience. Are your palms sweaty? Is your heart beginning to flutter? Is your stomach turning? Are you thinking, "Oh my, there are so many people out there," or worrying about what the crowd will think of you?

Whether it's a presentation, a playoff game, a life-threatening situation, or even a first date, performance under pressure is something we can all relate to. And here's a little secret: Paying attention to what you're thinking about is the first step to mastering your performance.

When we react to stress, sometimes the brain and body respond in a way that is not always best for the situation. One example is how stress impacts our attention. If you are in a room with a rattlesnake, you're likely not paying attention to the colour of the curtains! Biological programming locks your attention on the snake. This is what psychologists refer to as the "threat-rigidity response."

The downside is that sometimes we don't want our attention to become narrow and rigid. Think of how important it is for an advertising executive to be able to think broadly and openly even when a deadline is approaching. Sometimes we want our attention to be flexible instead of focusing only on what we perceive to be our largest threat. Possessing the ability to stay calm under pressure is the bedrock of outstanding performance, because in a calm state we can more reliably regulate our attention and behaviour.

When we feel stressed out, simply taking deeper breaths for about 60 seconds can be very calming. Deep breathing activates the parasympathetic response in the body, which floods the brain with oxygen and signals to the emotional centres of the brain that it's time to de-stress.

If you consider highly stressful situations you've experienced at work, for example, you may be able to identify when pausing to take some deep breaths could have helped to calm your mind and open it to several possible solutions. That's where mindfulness can take you—to a today and tomorrow where you can achieve a state of calm and effectiveness at a higher level than ever before.

A simple mindfulness protocol to enhance focus and attention
With practice and time, your mindfulness training will begin to elicit remarkable results. You will start to notice when you are

distracted, which sounds simple but can be challenging for some people. It will put a stop to ruminating thoughts and help you stay in the moment, which is critical to performing at your best. My colleague and dear friend Dr. Ellen Choi, assistant professor at the Ryerson University School of Business in Toronto, recommends getting started by practising *present moment awareness*.

Take a few minutes to do nothing but observe what's happening. Stop and notice your thoughts and feelings. What are you touching and how does it feel (cold, warm, hot, smooth, rough, soft, hard)? What can you see in terms of shape, colour, texture, distance, closeness? What sounds are close by and farther away, and can you identify them all? What smells are in the air (your cologne, a cup of coffee, someone's lunch)? What taste do you have in your mouth (sweet, sour, metallic, bitter)? What do you feel in your chest, stomach, or hands (tightness, heat, sweat)?

Then choose an anchor—any point of focus that connects you to the present. Your anchor may be your breath, or body sensations like the feeling of your feet on the floor, or the temperature of your hands. It could also be a mantra you're repeating in your mind, or even something in front of you that you can lock your gaze on. Set your anchor and return to it anytime your mind wanders.

Practise paying attention to your anchor for a few moments each day and you will develop your ability to stay present, develop focus, connect to your body, and learn to control your attention.

For those of you who are always on the go without a minute to spare, just taking 10 seconds to pause and actually notice your experience ("I am really angry/stressed out/annoyed right now") is a powerful way to begin the process of regulating thoughts and actions (the foundation mindfulness training is built upon).

Becoming aware of what's actually happening inside you is the first step to improving your performance.

This technique involves being 100% present in the moment, with all attention directed at one thing only. I can do this when I listen to a great piece of music. I also love art galleries—when faced with a masterpiece, it's difficult to think about anything else. Try this when in conversation with a friend or family member: Focus only on what they're saying. Don't let your mind wander or worry about what you're going to say back. You'll be amazed by the power of this technique. One of the deepest human needs is the desire to be listened to.

Sharpening your focus and living in the moment are great ways to dissipate stress. So much of our stress comes from thinking about the past or the future. When we stay in the present, we often

1% TIP: USE TECHNOLOGY TO PRACTISE MINDFULNESS

Mindfulness is another area of our lives where technology can be part of the problem *and* the solution. There are many tools available to help you incorporate mindfulness into your routine, such as the Headspace and Calm apps. Another option is Muse, which is a headband that picks up brain activity and works with an app to guide you into different brain states. While wearing it, you hear waves gently crashing on the beach. As soon as your mind begins to wander, the band picks up the mental activity and changes the sound to storms. The stormy sounds are your cue to refocus. Once you go more than 30 seconds with no change in brain activity, the sound changes to birds tweeting and points are awarded.

realize that things are pretty good. Practise for a few moments each day and you will develop your ability to stay present, focus, connect to your body, and control your attention.

Key #2 (Body): Energize Your Body to Engage Your Mind

A few years ago, Dr. Isabelle Senécal came to my lab for a research placement. In addition to being a clinician, she was a high-level soccer referee. She wanted to explore how fatigue and exercise intensity affected decision-making ability in elite soccer referees.

Dr. Senécal recruited some referees and put them through their paces on a treadmill. While running, the refs would perform the Stroop Test to check on the speed and accuracy of their cognitive performance. (In a Stroop Test, participants see how fast they can complete mental tasks and how many errors they make as they run to exhaustion.) We hypothesized that as the referees became fatigued, they would make more mistakes.

We could not have been more wrong. Performance on the Stroop Test improved at submaximal and maximal exercise intensities! The referees answered questions more quickly and with no change in the number of errors made. Dr. Senécal suggested that the referees were able to focus their attention to improve their "goal-oriented processing" during physical exertion. The harder the referees exercised, the more they were able to focus and the better they got at the cognitive tests.

How can those of us who are not professional baseball players or elite referees leverage movement to help us focus better?

Growing research shows that physical activity improves brain function and facilitates learning, creativity, and problem-solving, among other key functions. Even simple movements like walking before a mental task can help you do that task better. Researchers in Japan discovered that a short bout of moderate-intensity exercise (at 50% of a person's maximum intensity) improved reaction time on the Stroop Test after the exercise session ended. Similar research subsequently performed by another group in Japan showed that improvements in cognition (speed and accuracy) were demonstrated at 40% of maximum intensity, with an increase in cognitive performance matched by improvements in blood flow and oxygenation of the brain.

Even better: Jeffrey Miller and Zlatan Krizan from Iowa State University found that short bouts of exercise not only help with your mental processing, memory recall, and accuracy, but also improve your mood and make you feel more energetic.

Increasing focus isn't just about aerobic activity. Yoga has long been known as a practice that emphasizes mind–body–energy connections. In fact, an overwhelming amount of research supports the notion that yoga does indeed improve our health and performance. In a recent review article, professor Tanvi Bhatt and his team in the Department of Physical Therapy at the University of Illinois at Chicago concluded that breathing, meditation, and posture-based yoga increased overall brainwave activity and helped to improve the function of the amygdala, which is involved in processing the experience of emotions and the activation of the frontal cortex of the brain. The frontal cortex is thought to help with skeletal movement, movement of the eyes, speech, and the expression of emotion.

The overall increase in brainwave activity may explain the decreases in anxiety and increases in focus that are evident after yoga training programs. Overall, yoga seems to have positive effects on brainwave activity in terms of stimulating the activation of alpha, beta, and theta brainwaves, which have been associated with improvements in cognition, memory, mood, and anxiety.

An exercise protocol to help you focus better and more easily
We know that if we have an important mental task to do, a 15-minute walk, jog, or bike ride beforehand can help us focus and perform. We'll feel better, have more energy, and think more quickly and accurately. Yoga or even just some deliberate deep-breathing exercises beforehand can also help.

That's just a single bout of exercise. What would happen if we did this consistently over time? How would that change our brain and our ability to control our attention, focus, and maybe even prevent age-related cognitive decline?

Dr. Arthur Kramer's lab at the University of Illinois specializes in trying to answer those questions. In a series of studies, they found that cardiorespiratory endurance—how fit our heart, lungs, blood, and muscles are—has a positive effect on our brain function, and that better cardiorespiratory fitness is related to better outcomes in people with neurodegenerative disorders. They have also shown that 6 months of exercise training changes the brain and stimulates growth and better activation of the frontal and temporal lobes, along with the hippocampus.

Add some cardio to your weekly plan and stick with it. Your brain will thank you! Three to five sessions a week (walking, jogging, swimming, biking, paddling, or spinning) that last anywhere from 15 to 45 minutes will keep every organ in your body working better, not just in moments when you need to focus and perform, but for the rest of your life as well.

1% TIP: HAVE FUN GETTING OUT THERE

In this book I've talked a lot about the importance of exercise for controlling focus and attention, in addition to the major benefits it has on our physical health, but exercise is also essential for establishing and sustaining a joyful and positive mood. And when you are in a good mood, it's much easier to perform at your best.

Done properly, exercise feels good: It makes your brain work better, it improves your attention, it amplifies your performance, it gives you confidence, and it makes you happier. The benefits will be immediate and long-lasting.

Finding joy in movement will keep you motivated to exercise. If you are struggling to exercise consistently, just commit to doing 5 minutes. Put on your gear and get out there. If after 5 minutes you want to stop, that's fine. But I doubt you will.

Key #3 (Space): Harness the Power of Cold

The use of cold therapy has a very long history. Hippocrates, the father of the field of medicine, is said to have prescribed cold baths for his patients to alleviate "lassitude" (physical and mental fatigue). The effects of cold exposure have been of growing interest for researchers and practitioners, although there is still a lot of debate and work needed to really tease out what is going on physiologically when we come into contact with cold air or cold water.

We do know that several effects occur when we expose ourselves to cold. The very first thing that happens, especially when we come into contact with cold water, is a rapid cardiorespiratory response to the cooling of the skin that triggers a gasping response and inhalation of 1 to 2 litres of air. If your face is below the surface of the water when this happens, then of course drowning is very likely.

If you manage to actually immerse yourself in the cold water, the next physiological response is a reduction in tissue temperature, which subsequently affects blood flow, cell swelling, and metabolism as well as how fast your nerves can communicate with each other. This is what athletes who sit in cold tubs after training or games are trying to achieve. Muscle temperature decreases when the body is immersed in 10°C water that is at least 30 millimetres deep for at least 10 minutes. Systemically, cold therapy not only causes our core temperature to reduce, but induces cardiovascular and endocrine changes as well. Placing the body in cold water up to the waist or in some cases to the chest or neck is now known in the scientific literature as cold-water immersion (CWI).

CWI is known to activate the sympathetic nervous system, increase the blood level of beta-endorphins, and increase the release of noradrenaline in the synapses of the neurons of the brain. Beta-endorphins are known to produce feelings of euphoria, regulate the reward systems in the brain, and help to diminish activity in areas of the brain related to stress—the same effects produced by running and meditation. Basically, cold water might be able to give you the sensation of a "runner's high" without the running!

While taking an ice bath might not seem like a practice you want to adopt, a cold shower might be a powerful option for you. Due to the high density of cold receptors in the skin, a cold shower can trigger increased electrical impulses from peripheral nerve endings to the brain, which could result in a number of physiological effects in the body and the brain. This can help with the release of adrenaline, which has been shown to improve concentration, focus, and alertness for hours afterward.

Dutch researcher Dr. Geert Buijze conducted a study where he and colleagues asked 3,000 volunteers in the Netherlands to finish their morning showers with a 30- to 90-second blast of cold water. They then compared the data collected against the results from people who took their normal morning showers. They found that the cold-shower group reported 29% fewer sick days than the regular shower group. They also noticed that if the cold-shower group exercised, they experienced 54% fewer sick days. The researchers were clear that they did not examine the mechanisms of the effects, but they hypothesized that cold water activates our stress "fight or flight response," which causes the release of cortisol and adrenaline into the system, which in turn may increase the activity of the immune system for short periods of time.

Interestingly, it's not just physiology that appears to adapt to cold-water exposure. In a recent case report, researchers described a 24-year-old woman with symptoms of major depressive disorder and anxiety who had been treated for the condition since the age of 17. Following the birth of her daughter, she wanted to be medication- and symptom-free. She adopted a program of weekly open cold-water swimming. Within a month, she was able to reduce her medication; after 4 months, she no longer required drug treatment. On follow-up a year later, she remained medication-free. Was her improvement due to the cold or the swimming?

We're not sure, but the results are compelling. More research is needed to bring clarity to the use of cold for people with mental-health challenges.

Before you jump into an ice-cold bath or take a cold shower, keep in mind that cold-water exposure does not necessarily feel good. Your body can't really differentiate between cold and pain, so you might perceive the cold as painful. It will, however, make you mentally tough. Once you've had an ice-cold shower to start your day, everything else just seems easy.

Three cold-immersion protocols to help you improve focus
Cold-water exposure is a great opportunity to work on your ability to control your attention and focus. While you are exposed to cold water, breathe slowly. Concentrate on the moment. Over time, this will get easier and easier. Here are a few strategies to get you started:

1. **Take a cold bath.** If you want to go all in on cold-water immersion, you can install a cold tub in your home. Or you can just take a bath with cold water and some ice. You only need to do it once or twice a week to reap the rewards. To activate your immune system and focus your mind, try 5 minutes in cold (10°C) water followed by 5 minutes in air (that is, step out of the bath for a bit), and then repeat the cycle a second time.

2. **Finish your morning shower with a short blast of cold water.** Cold-water exposure is a great way to supercharge your morning. It can have an effect with as little as 20 or 30 seconds of exposure, so you can simply finish off your morning shower with a jolt of water as cold as you

can tolerate. Over time, you can build up to less time in warm water and more time in the cold shower.

3. **Set the thermostat.** It's not just cold water that you can leverage. A work environment that is too hot or too cold can impact your attention and focus. Research from Cornell University found that people are most productive and make the fewest errors in temperatures between 20°C and 25°C. A similar study by scientists in Finland suggested that the magic temperature for working on mental tasks is 22°C. Check your room temperature and make adjustments, if you can.

A word of caution: Be careful with cold exposure and alternating between hot and cold temperatures. If you do it wrong, it can kill you. When you are in cold water and breathing deeply, for example, there is a danger that you may blow off your carbon dioxide (which makes the blood vessels in your brain shrink) and pass out. There is also the "cold shock" response, which is very dangerous. Be safe and make sure you are not alone when you practise CWI therapy. Also, note that immersion in water under

---

1% TIP: UNLOCK RADICAL ATTENTION

I believe that a prerequisite of high performance is the ability to refocus with laser precision and total immersion on one thing at a time when your mind is wandering. That's how we unlock our ability to truly experience life at the highest possible level in each and every moment. Keep practising and this will get easier and easier.

15°C can cause hypothermia. I'd strongly recommend spending no more than 5 to 10 minutes doing any of the protocols listed above. Before you try anything, check with your doctor to make sure that CWI is safe for you.

Key #4 (Practice): Be Actively Engaged

We are in the early days of the internet revolution, an era of constant and unrelenting distraction. We are 10 years into something that will drastically change the way we live and work for the next 100 years. Not unlike when the world shifted from agriculture to industry, we are now shifting from industry to technology.

With the prevalence of smartphones, it seems everyone is expected to constantly check their email, even after work hours. We are never out of reach. We never unplug. And we are paying for the constant distraction mentally, physically, and emotionally.

The widespread addiction to distraction and all it entails—including the incessant inundation of text messages, social media, television, and email—has the potential to cause mental-health challenges. In fact, the overload we face every day and the seemingly endless stream of notifications are significant contributors to anxiety. The constant distraction leads to higher levels of distress and leaves us feeling burned out and exhausted.

The simple act of sitting down to focus on one task is becoming increasingly difficult for most people. Distraction is destroying our ability to do our best work on the things that matter most to us, whether it's career, school, business, or our most important relationships.

In his book *The Five Thieves of Happiness*, Dr. John Izzo articulates a way of thinking about technology use that can help us manage distraction: passive consumption versus active engagement. Izzo explains that passive consumption is scrolling through your feed, constantly observing other people and how great their life looks based on the perfection portrayed in their Instagram and other media posts. No one posts failures. They don't share pics of themselves when they wake up in the morning and their hair is all over the place. They don't share their reaction when they realize they made a big mistake. People post successes, vacations, and perfect selfies.

If you are constantly exposed to stories of perfect lives, your mental health will be negatively affected. Passive engagement is a form of distraction that not only erodes our ability to focus when we want and need to, but also leads to a less-than-healthy mental state.

Active engagement is different. If you use social media in a controlled and limited way to share celebrations, congratulate each other, offer encouragement, or ask questions about what people are up to, it can be an inspiring form of connection. If used *deliberately*, it can improve and support your mental health because it enables you to create a community around you.

Use technology to enhance your ability to do what you love better—ideally without experiencing any negative health effects. Connect with people to build deeper, stronger relationships. In some cases, that may mean using FaceTime to video call your kids while you're travelling. Other times, it means putting your phones away at dinner so you can have a face-to-face conversation. The point is to use technology with intention, *not* compulsion.

Use your deep focus for key things you want to accomplish. Allow yourself time to scan social media and relax. Then refuel and recharge so you are ready for your next important moment.

Exercise Your Brain

Your brain is constantly adapting and changing based on what you are doing and what is going on in your environment. Binge-watching Netflix? Your brain is adapting—maybe not for the better. Reading a biography of an epic historical figure? Your brain is adapting—probably for the better. Building on this idea, here are a few ways you can exercise your brain:

- **Hold walking meetings.** Have something you need to talk to someone about? Try talking while walking, rather than sitting across the table from each other. You can also do walking phone calls. Changing your environment, physical exercise, and navigating all help to improve brain function.
- **Play games.** Have some fun playing Sudoku, chess, or role-playing games, or just do a crossword puzzle. Your brain will thank you.
- **Learn something new.** When I was getting ready to commentate on the Olympics, I took acting and voice lessons. As an athlete and academic, I can tell you that was *way* out of my comfort zone. And I loved it. Learning something new at any age is powerful and can spark new cognitive abilities. Change up your reading list, take a dance lesson, pick up a new instrument, or try a new sport.

WORDS OF WISDOM: DR. BRYNN WINEGARD ON THE DOPAMINE FEEDBACK LOOP

Dr. Brynn Winegard is an award-winning professor, speaker, and world-leading expert on the intersection of business and brain science.

Our brains have synapses that run on dopamine, which is now understood to be the "action" neurochemical. It's basically the brain's reward for having done something that it wanted to do. It interacts with our brains' neuroplasticity because when you do something and receive a positive response, internally even, your brain will want to do it again. It will lay down pathways for wanting to do it again. You just have to choose how you will apply that feedback loop. If you allow it to operate on a non-functional habit, like smoking, it will reinforce the behaviour and you become addicted. Whereas, if you allow it to work on a functional habit, like exercise, it will recur and enhance your health.

THE TAKEAWAY ON RADICAL ATTENTION AND DELIBERATE RECHARGING

History is packed with amazing people whose accomplishments came partly from the ability to continuously learn and grow. It's doubtful they were born with some sort of superpower. In fact, my guess is that they experimented with life tweaks—including what we might call mental and physical health adjustments—until they found a formula that worked for them. Some of them got up early—not to pack their days more tightly but to free up morning or evening time for personal and leisure activities. Some of them were night owls, for the same reason. Many—from Beethoven to Emerson to Einstein—punctuated their days with exercise. Others blocked out time for reflection or meditation. Gandhi was known for his baths, massages, and long walks. You get the idea.

Cultivating a passion for life and maintaining our ability to be engaged and to grow means intentionally activating our mental focus and performing at our best, but then alternating those periods of intense concentration with moments—or hours or days or weeks—to reflect and recharge. We can't stay in an alert, activated state at all times. We will only damage our minds and bodies through overwork or overactivation (in relation to our focus and beta state).

Remember the five sacrifices (see page 3)? Four of them are linked to a perpetually overactivated state: giving up health for wealth, quality for quantity, response-ability for reaction, and internal motivation for external rewards. The fifth names a culprit that steals away our focus when we really need it: sacrificing attention for distraction. To reach the heights of which we're all capable—to be our own version, in our own way, of the contemporary or historical greats we admire—we need to take our mental abilities seriously and cultivate them sensibly, to be stewards and not just users of our minds and bodies. This means taking action against the world in some ways. Because let's be honest: This is a world that sends us messages to go faster, do more, keep connected, and stay busy. Don't listen to these messages! They're dangerous.

Instead, use the science of performance to upgrade your life, elevate your wellness, boost your energy, and unlock your potential.

Focus fully and deeply when you ought to—to bring your dreams to fruition. Recharge fully and deeply when you ought to—to nourish and sustain both that focus and those dreams.

Radical attention to perform. Deliberate regeneration to recharge. This strategy changes life from a marathon to a series of fun sprints interspersed with moments of recovery and recharging. That's the key to sustainable high performance and improved health.

STEP 4: DO LESS
(TO ACHIEVE MORE)

"A busy calendar and a busy mind will destroy your ability to do great things in this world. If you want to be able to do great things, whether you're a musician, or whether you're an entrepreneur, or whether you're an investor, you need free time and you need a free mind."
—Naval Ravikant

Newness comes into the world through creativity and imagination. This is true of all fields: science as much as poetry, entrepreneurship as much as fashion, sports as much as business. If we can't see past *what is* to *what could be*, then we cannot create something that currently doesn't exist. We can't find a new solution, build a better team, design a more effective medical treatment, even anticipate our own future growth. In a creative state, our mind is open, curious, and spontaneous.

Maybe you're doubtful about the value of creativity—maybe you see it as a requirement for writing a novel or a symphony but not so relevant to your life or work. I would respectfully submit that creativity, ideation, and agile thinking are absolutely crucial for us as we craft a beautiful life. Remember Einstein's words: "I am enough of the artist to draw freely upon my imagination. Imagination is more important than knowledge. Knowledge is limited. Imagination encircles the world."

Creativity is so vital to success that a recent IBM Global CEO study identified creativity as the most important leadership quality. The Boston Consulting Group has been running an annual strategy survey since 2011. For 7 out of the 8 years between 2011 and 2019, creativity and innovation were the top-ranked strategic imperatives. There's a similar emerging emphasis in education: Learning environments need to focus less on the transmission of knowledge and more on developing capabilities that will see students through all types of learning and leading situations—critical thinking, communication, collaboration, and creativity.

With creativity at such a premium in our fast-paced and rapidly changing world, scientists are increasingly interested in how to amplify it. In one recent experiment, Elisabeth Hertenstein at the University of Freiburg, Germany, and her colleagues used a technology called *transcranial direct current stimulation* (TDCS) to see if they could stimulate creativity. Electrodes attached to the scalp passed a tiny current through the brain, with the positive electrode stimulating brain cells on the right side of the inferior frontal gyrus (an area associated with problem-solving) and the negative electrode placed on the left side. The idea was to increase activity on the right side, which tends toward more out-of-the-box freethinking, and reduce it on the left. The result? Students performed 10% to 20% better on three creative tasks compared to others with "sham" electrodes without any electrical current.

This kind of scientific interest speaks to the value of creativity in all walks of life. Consider that quite often the biggest moments in our lives are those when we put the most pressure on ourselves: sitting down to write a university entrance exam, waiting to be interviewed for a dream job, or asking someone to go on a date for the first time. These moments happen at critical junctures, and the outcomes can change the trajectory of our entire lives.

To ensure that we are able to ask the right questions, to perform to our potential in the moment, to remember the key facts, or to create a new insight, we need to make sure that we don't fall into tension (the typical reaction) but rather that we relax so we can enter into the state we need to be in for whatever task it is that we want to do.

1% TIP: THE CHEMICAL COCKTAIL FOR CREATIVITY

Professor Baba Shiv from the Graduate School of Business at Stanford University studies the role that neural structures in the brain play in the biological roots of creativity. Dr. Shiv has suggested that creativity is achieved when there is a balance between the neurotransmitters serotonin (involved in regulating the sensations of calm and contentment versus anxiety and fear) and dopamine (which influences our shift from boredom and apathy to excitement and engagement). The ideal conditions for creativity might be high levels of both serotonin and dopamine, where we are calm but energized.

PIVOT FROM TENSION TO IDEATION

I've spent a lot of time trying to crack the code of ultra-performance. I've been looping back through everything I've learned as a scientist and physiologist, and comparing it to everything I am learning from meeting and working with some of the highest-achieving people on the planet. What I've observed is that elite performers are able to achieve a state of being where they can access their full potential. One of the best examples I can think of is Alex Honnold.

Honnold is the greatest free solo climber of all time. He climbs some of the most challenging rock faces in the world without any safety equipment at all. No ropes. No harness. Just his shoes, a chalk bag, and his unprecedented abilities. On June 3, 2017, after years of intense preparation, Honnold accomplished what many argue is one of the greatest athletic feats of all time: the first free solo ascent of a face of a massive rock outcropping in Yosemite called El Capitan. It took him 3 hours and 56 minutes. The entire odyssey of Honnold's preparation, including the climb itself, was captured in the Academy Award–winning documentary *Free Solo* by two of his close friends, wife and husband team Elizabeth Chai Vasarhelyi and Jimmy Chin.

When the climb had just been completed, videographer Jimmy Chin said some interesting things about Honnold:

> *Alex's process to prepare for his dream of free soloing El Cap has been an incredible, and sometimes stressful, journey to witness and be a part of . . . I expected (and prayed for) nothing less on his big day, but it was still mind-bending to see how relaxed he was in the final days leading*

up to the climb and of course during the climb . . . What I've learned over the last 10 years about Alex is he isn't the kid that shows up to do well on the exam. If it counts, he's there to ace it, knock out the extra-credit questions, and finish early. I'd say he aced his final exam yesterday with extra credit for style and composure. When he got to the top, he looked at me and said, "I'm pretty sure I could go back to the bottom and do it again right now." Congrats, bud. You crushed. It was historic, it was brilliant, it was moving beyond words.

The fact that Honnold found it only moderately challenging is fascinating. He prepared so much that one of the greatest athletic accomplishments in human history was almost easy.

While so much of what Honnold accomplished is hard for us to relate to, I think that Honnold's story is consistent with other great performers across various disciplines: They have the ability to stay relaxed while performing so they can access their true potential and be fully creative in the moment.

It's widely accepted that stress in the mind can lead to stress in the body, but the reverse is also true: Stress in the body can compromise the mind. That's why tension is a problem for creativity. Tension consumes energy inefficiently and decreases circulation, leading to physical aches and pains. When you achieve a relaxed state, however, you can get relief from aches and pains and improve digestion, cardiovascular function, and sleep—all of which will improve your mental performance and allow you to access your creativity in those moments when you most need it. Maybe it's when you're stuck on a problem or when something isn't working at the office. Maybe you need to change direction in life so you can have exceptional experiences and realize your dreams. For any and all of those "maybes" to happen, you need to pivot from tension to ideation.

So how can we make that shift, especially in the too fast, too crowded lives we tend to lead?

Practise Conscious Relaxation

If you tense your muscles for long periods of time, you will begin to feel the effects of that tension in your body and your mind. Your muscles hurt. Your patience wears thin. You become mentally fatigued. Your creativity goes out the window. Experiment with this by clenching your fists and paying attention to the physical and mental effects. You will feel the muscle tension triggering stressful thoughts.

Remember, the mind–body link runs both ways, so releasing tension from the body frees the mind from strain and pressure and leads to a state of relaxation and improved ideation. This is a critical physical and mental skill you can learn and use. For example, practise *tension to relaxation* to stop yourself from bracing, which is a habit of lifting your shoulders and clenching your muscles. To accomplish this, begin by becoming aware of muscle tightness and body position. Ask yourself the following questions:

1. Can I drop my shoulders?
2. Can I relax my hands? Stomach? Legs? Forehead?
3. Can I sit in a more comfortable position?
4. Can I relax my core and deepen my breathing?

When you find an area of tension, breathe in and out deeply and slowly to release the tension. Let go of tightness, pressure, and fatigue.

A deeper practice technique is called *progressive relaxation*, which consists of alternating 3 to 5 seconds of tension with 10 to 15 seconds of relaxation of various muscle groups:

1. Sit in a chair, lean back, and make yourself comfortable.
2. Close your eyes.
3. Lift your toes as high as possible. Hold. Release and let the tension go into the floor. Point your toes. Repeat.
4. Tense the upper part of your legs. Hold. Relax. Feel your legs against the chair and your feet against the floor. Experience the relaxation.
5. Tighten your stomach muscles . . . then relax. Take a deep breath. Feel the tension in your chest. Exhale and relax. Concentrate on how calm you can get.
6. Make tight fists with your hands and hold for about 5 seconds. Unclench your hands and let the tension flow out, noting how it feels different to relax.
7. Do the same with your upper arms, then your neck. Frown, and then relax. Take a moment to notice any other areas of tension and concentrate on releasing those as well.
8. Take a few deep breaths and open your eyes. Or keep them closed. Either way, you will have released your tension and created a quiet, peaceful space for creativity.

Awareness of your body is key to pivoting from tension to ideation. The more you practise these relaxation techniques, the easier they are to use and the easier it becomes to tap into your creative potential. Imagine how a painter could do beautiful work

WORDS OF WISDOM: ARIEL GARTEN ON HOW TO BE CALM IN THE MOMENT

Ariel Garten is a neuroscientist and psychotherapist who is at the forefront of the emerging field of brain-sensing technology. Ariel is co-founder of InteraXon, a startup that developed the Muse meditation headband.

You can relax your physiology in real time by breathing deeply or stretching a little beforehand. Deep breaths significantly change your physiology. As you breathe out, your heart rate slows. You can also focus on addressing your amygdala to reassure your system that the situation is not dangerous, that there is no need to freak out. Or you can focus on remembering a time when you felt calm and then just let that feeling seep throughout your entire body. Anything to shift the focus away from the fear toward physiological calm, physiological safety, and physiological relaxation. And, of course, you can also change the way you perceive energy you experience. Instead of choosing to view it as nervousness and stress, you can see it as excitement and channel the energy into your performance.

The real blue sky for me is if everyone in the world meditated and had a real practice, and through doing and building the empathy and compassion that meditation builds, we would have world peace. I know that sounds super far out there, but when you kind of walk back the logic on it, the reason that we have war, the reason that you invade another land, is fear. If everybody was able to increase their levels of compassion and empathy, if everybody was able to reduce their fear, anxiety, and scarcity thinking, the world would be a pretty peaceful place.

in a relaxed, creative state compared to when they are tired and tense. The same goes for musicians, athletes, students, parents, and business leaders.

A breathing protocol to help you relax quickly

Stress, agitation, negative emotion, and busyness are the biggest threats to accessing your zone. When tension creeps into your calm yet high-energy, high-output zone state, your effort increases but your performance drops. You get tight and you start to fight to stay in the zone.

Because the centres of your brain that control breathing are closely linked to the area that controls stress, breathing is an effective way to combat stress. If you can calm the electrical activity in the breathing centre, then you have a good chance of calming the stress, which is why yoga and meditation work.

Deep, controlled breathing to calm anxiety or stress is often called *combat breathing*. You can practise combat breathing any-time you feel that you are slipping out of your zone or having trouble getting into it. Here's how:

1. Get into good posture by aligning your spine and stretch-ing yourself upward. You can be lying down, sitting in a chair, or standing.

2. Relax your muscles. Mentally scan your body and take note of any tension. Focus on that tense area while you take slow, deep breaths. Think about "letting go" of the tension as you exhale. (It might take a few breaths to get an area like your shoulders or forehead to release and relax.)

3. Once you feel you have addressed the tense areas, start taking controlled breaths. (I usually inhale for 4 seconds, hold it for 2 seconds, and then exhale for 6 seconds.)

The point is to realize you are stressed and then take slow, deep breaths. This will help you let go of stress no matter what you are preparing for—a presentation, a performance, a competition, an exam, anything.

Act-Think-Feel

Athletes use rituals to help themselves calm down in moments of tension. They know that tension, stiffness, and worry are toxic for a great performance. Olympic snowboarder Jamie Anderson hugs trees before her key runs. She also uses a pre-competition meditation ritual to stay calm and focused. Olympic cyclist Laura Kenny brings her attention to her breath and deliberately relaxes her muscles to help minimize her anxiety before competing: "It sounds stupid but by thinking about your breathing, it stops you thinking about anything else. If you push your belly out when you take a breath in, like doing the opposite to what you think you should do, it really helps." Michael Phelps practised visualization and rehearsed many different circumstances and how he would deal with them. He knew what he would do if his suit ripped or his goggles broke. This helped him stay calm and confident in the moment.

By calming down their bodies and brains, athletes are able to align their thoughts and feelings to the state they need to be in to perform at their best. I call it "Act–Think–Feel."

The basic physiology is simple: If you move your body or think in a particular way, you signal your body to release hormones that change the way you think and feel. For example, Jared Martin and Dr. Paula Niedenthal at the University of Wisconsin–Madison have reported that deliberately smiling can help decrease levels of the stress hormone cortisol after public speaking faster than other facial expressions. Further, the neurotransmitters that make you feel good—dopamine, endorphins, and serotonin—are all released when you smile. Simply, we can use our bodies to influence our minds, and vice versa.

The challenge is that Act–Think–Feel is not the typical sequence we go through when we are under pressure. Usually, negative emotions like fear, nervousness, or anger come first and then create negative thoughts that lead to poor performance and poor outcomes. Usually, the order is Feel–Think–Act. Just think of when something happened and you felt that sinking feeling in your stomach, got upset, and reacted by saying or doing something you later regretted. But we can create a more positive and effective way of living if we deliberately use our knowledge of physiology. Remember, Act–Think–Feel.

I do my best to use the Act–Think–Feel technique to get into the state that I need to be in to perform, any time I want, rather than just having it "happen." The more I use this, the better I'm getting at using it in key moments. I'm not perfect, but it is definitely helping, and I'm getting better at it. For example, I like to use this technique if I'm speaking at an event and someone in the audience asks me a question that I don't know the answer to. With 1,000 people watching me think, the pressure can climb quickly. In moments like these, I try really hard to consciously relax, listen carefully, consider the question, and then answer as clearly as I can (and quickly admit I don't know the answer if I am still drawing a blank, which happens!).

Here's how you can control your physiology to activate your creativity:

1. Think about the last time you felt relaxed and at your best.
2. Figure out what you were *doing* before that moment. What were your actions? Were you stretching? Did you have a good breakfast? Write it down. This is the "Act."
3. Now figure out what you were *thinking*. Were you listening to a podcast or to music? Did you tell yourself what you were going to do? What mindset did you have? This is the "Think."
4. Remember what you were *feeling*. What were your emotions? How did they help you to relax? This is the "Feel."

You'll end up with a road map for the same kind of process that elite athletes go through when they're preparing for an event. Then the next time you're faced with a moment that triggers your stress response and mental and physical tension, you'll know exactly the physical state you need to be in (Act) so you can give yourself the best chance of having the right thoughts in that moment (Think), and then create the emotional state you need

> **1% TIP: IMPROVE YOUR LONGEVITY BY WALKING**
>
> There are just so many benefits to walking, and it's so easy to incorporate into your life. Studies have shown that walking can lower your risk of high blood pressure and diabetes, and is also associated with a reduced risk for over 12 different types of cancer. As little as 15 minutes of walking can improve longevity and even make you happier! Just get started and build it into your routine. Go for a walk after dinner, do a walking meeting, or go for a stroll with a friend.

to be in (Feel) to execute the task, build the relationship, hit the shot, make the decision, or perform the piece. As with most things, you'll get better at this with practice!

DO LESS TO ACCOMPLISH MORE— THETA BRAINWAVES

States where the brain exhibits theta brainwaves (see page 19) allow us to unleash our creativity and are enabled and enhanced by physical activity and rhythmic repetitive movements like walking, cycling, and taking in the patterns in nature (for example, leaves on a tree or a flock of birds flying by). Perhaps a more relatable situation is being on autopilot in the shower, going through the motions without thought, and having a new, seemingly random, idea pop into your mind.

Not surprisingly, theta brainwaves are similar to the delta brainwaves that happen during sleep. They occur at 4 to 7 cycles per second (Hz), whereas delta brainwaves cycle at 0.1 to 3 Hz. These are both slow-brainwave states.

I believe that deliberately moving into a creative state where we can ideate—characterized by theta brainwaves—is essential for unlocking our ability to reach our potential. We need to come up with new solutions to old problems: new ideas, new products, new or deeper relationships, and new opportunities. We can do this by relaxing our bodies, moving our bodies, and letting our brains make new connections and come up with new ideas.

When we are in a creative, problem-solving state characterized by theta wave activity, several regions of our brain activate at the same time and connect to each other. This is how we have leaps

WORDS OF WISDOM: DR. ELLEN CHOI ON HOW TO CALM YOUR MIND

Dr. Ellen Choi's research interests revolve around the effects of mindfulness training on attention, emotional regulation, and performance under pressure. She is currently an assistant professor at Ryerson University's School of Business.

If meditation scares you or makes you feel uncomfortable, or you just feel too busy to rest and slow down, then simply sitting quietly is where you can start. Whether it's for 1 minute or 5 minutes or 10 minutes, it really doesn't matter. To really savour and connect with what stillness feels like, we have to learn to stop and be still without associating it with boredom or inefficiency. You can increase the amount of time you spend in stillness as your comfort level grows.

For people who are new to meditation, I typically recommend meditating in the morning, because as the day gets busier, it becomes harder to overcome the inertia and slow down. The research supports the idea that starting in the morning is your best shot at getting this practice inculcated into your day.

To begin, I suggest committing to 3 minutes—that's like a long elevator ride or a walk to the printer. You can either set the timer on your phone for 3 minutes or just use a watch and open your eyes occasionally to see if 3 minutes has passed.

Then sit in a comfortable position, close your eyes, and choose a mental anchor. It can be a phrase, your breath, or a visualization of something that is important or meaningful for you (like a beach, a person, or a pursuit that you love). Just choose one thing to focus on and sit quietly, breathe, and try to hold onto that one thought.

Inevitably, your mind will wander and that's okay. Be kind, curious, and compassionate. Don't beat yourself up if the mind wanders: However old you are, you have that many years of your mind wandering in default mode. Just notice it and then come back to the anchor. Of course, this sounds really simple, but for people who tend to ruminate or keep thinking about something over and over, it can be hard to let go. For people who tend to relive all of their most embarrassing moments, meditation is so nice because you're literally building the neural mechanisms to help you let go of things faster.

That's essentially it: Pick an anchor, notice when the mind wanders, let go of that other thought or feeling, direct your mind back to the anchor, and then move through that process again until the time you've set aside to meditate is up.

of insight, and discover links we didn't see before. Counterintuitively, it is only by doing less and entering a theta wave state that we can accomplish more.

THE KEYS TO RELAXATION, CREATIVITY, AND IDEATION

In today's fast-paced world, it can be hard to feel like slowing down is even an option. But slowing down doesn't have to mean giving up on reaching our goals or getting through our to-do lists. Slowing down can allow us to generate and tap into our energy reserves so we can fulfill our responsibilities and achieve our dreams. Granted, it isn't always easy to accomplish—especially when we are under pressure to get through everything on our list.

Slowing down requires us to avoid getting caught up in the speed of our environment and to leverage the power of the creative theta wave state that will set the stage for us to leap forward in new, different, and positive ways.

Here are four keys to help you slow down so you can be more creative, ideate, and problem-solve better, and ultimately fully access your human potential.

Key #1 (Brain): Meditate to Regenerate Your Brain

Over the last few years, I have been integrating meditation into my life in a deliberate and purposeful way. I have also been encouraging all of my athletes, clients, audiences, and readers to do the same. Why? Because it is one of the simplest, most powerful, most wonderful things you can do for yourself. It's also a scientifically proven method for improving the functioning of your brain and extending your lifespan: People who meditate regularly experience a 23% reduction in all-cause mortality, a 30% reduction in cardiovascular mortality, and a 51% reduction in rate of cancer mortality—that's huge!

When we rest while awake—like when we meditate or pause to gaze out the window—the body and the brain take advantage of the decrease in activity to refuel and reset. More specifically, pausing to rest during our waking hours gives our bodies and brains the break that they need to replenish, setting the stage for getting back into the higher activity states that we use to get things done. If you're already thinking "I don't even have time to take a short break," then consider that even 3 minutes of meditation has been shown to have powerful benefits. That's less than 0.2% of your day!

New research by Adrienne Taren from the Center for Neuroscience at the University of Pittsburgh has demonstrated that regular meditation helps to change the responses of a region of the brain called the *amygdala* to environmental events. Overall, these changes result in better emotional control both during the meditation and in the hours that follow. Dr. Sy Saeed from the East Carolina University Brody School of Medicine has reported that meditation improves mood, stress, and hormone levels and can reduce anxiety, pain, and depression. It is an incredible tool that will make a huge difference in your life.

When we meditate, we create something called *brain-derived neurotrophic factor* (BDNF), a protein that helps existing neurons in our nervous systems survive and supports the growth of new ones. Studies have shown that BDNF and meditation have a very specific impact on the part of the brain called *grey matter*. Grey matter refers to the areas of the brain that contain almost all of the neuronal cells responsible for controlling everything from muscles to sensory perception, memory, emotions, speech, and decision-making. Grey matter is what you use to process information.

(Jokes about smart people having lots of grey matter aren't actually that far off the mark!) Recent research at Harvard University shows that meditating a few times per week for as little as 8 weeks can increase the grey matter in the parts of the brain responsible for emotional regulation and learning. That means that as little as 2 months of meditation can change your brain!

White matter is the part of your brain that connects all of the grey matter nodes together. It's a lighter colour because it contains myelin, a fatty substance that protects all of the nerves there like the bark on a tree. White matter responds mainly to a steady diet of healthy fats (because brain matter is made up of fats). If you are out for dinner, dump dark-green olive oil all over your meal. Or go for other sources of wonderful fats: cold-water fish, organic nut butters, coconut and avocados, omega-3 eggs, cod liver oil, flax seeds, chia seeds, and hemp seeds. These nutrients have been shown to improve white matter, which will improve the transmission of signals across your brain.

If your brain were a transit system, the grey matter would be the stations and the white matter would be the tracks. You can improve the functioning of your brain by bulking up the processing centres and improving the efficiency of transmission between nodes. Basically, you can enable the trains of your transit system to hold more, travel faster, and leave more often. Meditate to grow grey matter; consume healthy fats to improve white matter.

A simple meditation protocol to help calm your mind
If you want to get healthier and reach your potential, meditation should become one of your fundamental daily practices (see the Words of Wisdom by Dr. Ellen Choi on page 128).

Each day in the summer, I try to get out first thing in the morning and spend 15 to 20 minutes in meditation down by the lake near my home. The water rolls in, the breeze blows, and I feel like I am far away from the city (even though I can turn my head and see the city skyline full of office towers and condominiums). The peaceful state I enter through meditation allows me to calm my mind, creates openness, and energizes me for the day ahead. As a result, I find my ability to think clearly amplified, and that I am able to solve problems more readily. Most of all, I reconnect to a state of deep happiness.

Find a spot for yourself. A space just for you. Choose a place where you can let your mind completely relax. Let go of the urgent demands of life, just for a while, and try to reconnect to yourself. You can use an app to help you, if you like. I sometimes use

1% TIP: ADD SOME EXERCISE TO YOUR MEDITATION

Our minds affect the health of our bodies, just as our bodies affect the health of our minds. There is a relatively simple tool you can use to activate your brain-body connection and amplify your performance: mental and physical training (MAP).

1. Complete 20 (or more) minutes of cardio. It can be any kind—dancing, walking, running, jogging, swimming, etc.
2. As soon as you finish your workout, sit down, close your eyes, and meditate for 10 (or more) minutes. Meditation is an effortful training practice that involves learning about the transient nature of

thoughts and thought patterns, and acquiring skills to recognize them without necessarily attaching meaning and/or emotions to them.

Researchers have found that the MAP training approach can have a significant positive impact on symptoms of various conditions, such as depression, and ruminating thinking patterns. Recent research on the MAP technique has also shown that it stimulates neurogenesis—the growth of new neurons in the brain. The neurogenesis seems to happen in the hippocampus, which is the part of the brain that helps with learning and the creation of memories. I am hopeful that MAP training could help people learn more effectively throughout their lives. MAP is an incredibly powerful technique—and one that is easy to adopt if you can take a half-hour to pause and add it to your days.

Headspace.com, but Calm.com is also very popular. Muse is also a very cool piece of technology (**choosemuse.com**) that can help you start your own meditation practice.

If you set aside some time every day, even briefly, you will notice an enormous impact on your physical, emotional, and mental health. If you want to try out meditation, you can find a video of me leading a short practice at **vimeo.com/225027428**.

Key #2 (Body): Slow Down and Heat Up

Using heat to speed healing is a practice that spans centuries and cultures. We see it today in Russian banyas, Indigenous peoples' sweat lodges, and Finnish saunas. Not only can saunas be used to rest and relax (as they have been for centuries), but sauna bathing is a powerful practice that has health benefits for your body and brain.

The data supporting the health benefits of regular heat exposure via sauna bathing is compelling. For example, a study by Dr. Jari Laukkanen of the University of Eastern Finland suggested that people who engaged in frequent sauna use had reduced risks of fatal cardiovascular events and all-cause mortality. The researchers also reported that people who took two to three saunas per week had better outcomes than those who took only one per week, and that four to seven saunas per week had the highest association with survival and longevity. Similar results were found when it came to time spent per sauna use: Longer exposures of 20 minutes or more appeared to be more protective (see page 138).

When we expose ourselves to heat by way of traditional saunas or infrared saunas, a number of physiological changes have been reported, including increased bioavailability of nitric oxide, which improves the flexibility of the walls of your blood vessels (the vascular endothelium); the production of heat shock proteins (powerful proteins in the body that have a host of beneficial effects when activated); immune and hormonal pathway alterations; and enhanced excretions of toxicants through increased sweating.

Heat exposure also appears to improve cardiovascular health. Setor Kunutsor from the Bristol Biomedical Research Centre in the U.K. tracked 1,628 people over 15 years and found that compared with people who took saunas once a week, those who took them two to three times weekly were 12% less likely to have a stroke. People who took saunas four to seven times a week reduced their risk for stroke by 62%. Of course, this is an observational study and cannot prove causality, but the data is compelling.

In addition to the cardiovascular benefits, there may be positive health effects for people with inflammatory conditions. A recent review that summarized research on traditional Finnish and infrared saunas reported on the many benefits of heat exposure for people with rheumatic diseases such as fibromyalgia, rheumatoid arthritis, and ankylosing spondylitis, as well as patients with chronic fatigue and pain syndromes, chronic obstructive pulmonary disease, and allergic rhinitis. When people with these health challenges took regular saunas (30 minutes at 73°C in 10% to 20% humidity), blood, arterial stiffness, and cardiovascular system markers were all observed to improve.

There also appear to be powerful benefits for the brain. Research indicates that repeated sauna exposure seems to decrease the risk of Alzheimer's disease and dementia. In addition, new research shows that, once the body has returned to baseline temperature after taking a sauna, some networks of neurons in the brain are more relaxed and some cognitive processes can be performed more efficiently. A lot more research is needed to tease out the effects of heat exposure on the brain, but these early results are interesting and exciting.

Heat exposure also helps with adaptation that improves athletic performance. Think of it as training while you sit and relax in a really hot room! Benefits include increased growth hormone levels, muscle regrowth after training, increased blood volume, and increased overall endurance. So if you are into sports or are training for an athletic event like a run or triathlon, saunas and heat exposure may be something to consider adding to your routine.

Note that although sauna bathing is safe for most people, there are risks. Contraindications to sauna bathing include unstable angina pectoris, recent myocardial infarction, and severe aortic

1% TIP: TAKE SAUNAS TO LENGTHEN YOUR LIFE

A growing body of research suggests a strong link between regular heat bathing—saunas, for example—and reduced risk of chronic disease and longer lifespans. Dr. Rita F. Redberg, a cardiologist at the University of California, San Francisco, and editor-in-chief of *JAMA Internal Medicine*, has explained that people who take saunas more frequently have greater longevity. Whether it is the time spent in the hot room, the relaxation time, the leisure of a life that allows for more relaxation time, or the camaraderie of the sauna that is responsible for longevity has yet to be determined.

stenosis. Check with your doctor to make sure saunas are safe for you. Also, alcohol consumption during sauna bathing increases the risk of hypotension, arrhythmia, and sudden death, so if you take a sauna, don't drink any alcohol!

A simple heat protocol to help you regenerate better

There is very good evidence that heat exposure can reduce the risk of mortality and has positive effects on cardiovascular system health. Heat exposure also seems to improve inflammation in the body and helps to prevent brain diseases. Saunas help people relax and can provide athletes with physiological gains that improve exercise performance. Simply put, I'm a fan. I think that you can give this a try and get some great benefits, too.

If you don't have a sauna, that's totally fine. Sit in a hot bath a couple of times a week. Water is very powerful at transferring heat and cold in and out of the body. There is a lot of discussion about whether steam, dry, or infrared saunas are best, but the data is inconclusive at this time.

In a perfect world, a daily practice would be great, but just add what you can to your week. Remember: There is a dose–response effect with heat exposure. Even one session per week has proven benefits.

In terms of time, consider what you can build into your busy life and stick with it consistently. Benefits have been shown with sessions that last less than 10 minutes, but there appear to be increased benefits at 11 to 19 minutes and even more at 20 to 29 minutes. Note that 30 minutes is the longest duration I recommend, mainly for safety reasons (see below).

When it comes to temperature, most conventional sauna heaters warm the air to between 70°C and 100°C, with an optimal temperature around 80°C at head level. Steam in saunas makes it harder to move heat out of the body and should be enjoyed at a lower temperature ranging from 60°C to 70°C. Infrared saunas operate at even lower temperatures than traditional saunas, typically ranging from 45°C to 60°C.

My favourite protocol is to spend 5 to 10 minutes in dry heat at 80°C and then 5 minutes in a cool shower. Basically, I sit in a sauna until I start sweating, have a cool shower, and then repeat the loop one to three times, depending on how much time I have that day.

Perhaps the most important thing to remember when it comes to sauna bathing is to rehydrate after your session. People can easily lose 0.5 kilograms or more of water (that's a lot of sweat), so post–sauna use, make sure to drink water and eat electrolyte-rich foods such as nuts and seeds, avocados, tomatoes, cooked spinach, and fish.

Keep in mind that when you're in the sauna or a hot bath, it won't necessarily feel great. Consider it an opportunity to practise meditation, focus, and psychological discipline. One last thing: Be careful. Heat exposure can be dangerous. Heat exhaustion and heat stroke are real possibilities when doing these protocols (as they are when exercising outside in hot conditions). Start at a low heat and gradually build up, and stay within safe temperatures (40°C to 80°C). Check with your doctor before trying a sauna, to make sure it's safe for you.

1% TIP: STAY SAFE IN THE HEAT

Exercise or working in the heat can be dangerous, so stay safe. Keep cool with light clothing, drink lots of cold water, and use sun protection. If you are sweating, consume some electrolytes with your water to keep you hydrated and prevent cramping.

Key #3 (Space): Leverage the Power of Solitude

Accessing the full extent of our ability to invent and innovate requires learning to trigger the creativity pathway of our minds, and often. One way to do this is to organize a space where you can be creative. Often, that is a place of solitude: a room of your own. Maybe you go there when you are writing. Maybe you go there with a partner when you are working on a report or project and need to hide out. Maybe you take your team there to be sequestered and explore possibilities (like the Beatles did in Abbey Road Studios). Whatever the case may be, take control of your space so you can stimulate the right kind of mental activity.

Thomas Edison was famous for his prolific capacity to invent and innovate. One of his techniques was to have a dedicated space where he could do his thinking. It had a bedroom so he could nap, a small kitchen so he could make some food, and a zone for creative work. He also established a culture where everyone in the organization understood that disturbing him was fireable—this was "Do Not Disturb" to the extreme.

My creative place is in Central America. No internet. Jungle and ocean everywhere you look. A house I can rent for my family. That's where my deep thinking takes place. That's where I recover and regenerate. But it's only for 2 weeks at a time. It doesn't address my ongoing need for a space that supports creativity.

When I heard Steve Wozniak talk about deep creativity, I made a decision to emulate Thomas Edison's "invention factory," Menlo Park, in my home. Edison had a dedicated space where he could work undisturbed, be creative, and ideate. My space is pretty simple. It's a room with everything I need: art on the walls that I find beautiful and stimulating; a concert poster signed by two brilliant musicians I adore; an amazing piece of artwork by Jane Waterhouse right beside my desk; comfortable furniture; a computer; access to inspiring music; and a view of the park outside if I need to stare into the trees. Whenever I need to do deep thinking, this is where I go. The space pulses with creative energy for me. And the more I go in there, the more my mind learns that this is the place it can run. I get more and more creative. Then I take those ideas and head out into the world, places where I am surrounded by people and can engage in the types of productivity and creativity that happen in a group.

A few ideas to help you create your ideation space

You might not be able to change the state of your building or access a room of your own, but you can make small changes to workspaces or rooms that will make a big difference. You don't have to spend a ton of money, either. Work with what you have to create a space more conducive to creativity. Here are five easy ways to improve your creative space:

1. **Standing or walking desks:** These are great if you are working on a project that doesn't require you to be isolated. Plus, employees can use them for phone calls or emails. You can also use bar stools at high tables, which are great for leaning on when having a conversation.

2. **Change of scenery:** When possible and appropriate, try to get away from your desk. Hold walking meetings to energize your mind and get some fresh air. Even moving a meeting off-site to a local coffee shop can get the blood flowing in a way that sitting around in the usual place can't.

3. **Meditation rooms:** Some progressive companies such as Deloitte and Google offer meditation rooms with comfortable chairs and background music. Employees can go in, close their eyes, and take a break in a very quiet place that fosters mindfulness. If no such space exists for you, create your own by putting on headphones, positioning your chair so it is facing away from the door, or finding a place in the building—maybe in a warehouse or meeting room—where you can go to disconnect.

4. **Natural light:** Lighting can play an important role in a workspace. Natural light is far better for people than fluorescent lighting. If you work in an office with fluorescent lighting, be sure to get exposed to natural full-spectrum light a few times each day (yet another reason to go for a quick recharge walk). In addition, introducing plants into an office environment improves physical and mental health.

5. **A creative space at home:** I encourage everyone to create a home space that enables you and your loved ones to rest, refocus, and recharge, setting you up to be able to do what you love. With more and more people working from home at least part of the time, it's crucial to create an environment that inspires you to pursue your passions. If you are a person who frequently works remotely, create a "road warrior" kit: Equip yourself with high-quality noise-cancelling headphones and a journal or other meditation medium—anything you need to be fully focused on your tasks. If you are into art, set up a studio. If music is your jam, then a music room could be amazing.

Your environment needs to support what you are trying to accomplish—in this case, accessing a relaxed mental state via a space that supports creativity once it's under way.

1% TIP: CREATE A POSITIVE ENVIRONMENT

Your environment has a huge effect on you. Ask yourself if everything around you is supporting your well-being. How is the space where you sleep? How close is your gym or wherever you exercise? What kind of food is in your kitchen? What media do you consume regularly? What are you reading? Who are you following on social media?

Then ask yourself the most important question: Who are the people around you? Look for people who elevate you, encourage you, and inspire you.

When you set yourself up for success, you'll be on your way to leading an amazing life.

Key #4 (Practice): Disappear into Motion

One of the most powerful ways to slow down a racing mind and spark a calmer approach to life is—counterintuitively—to move. Specifically, to move in a rhythmic and repetitive activity like walking, running, swimming, biking, or paddling. Rhythmic movement helps us change our state from one in which we feel like we are hustling and racing around (the beta state) to one where our minds settle down (the theta state). When we do this with intention, I call it "moving meditation."

Moving meditation is any activity where your muscles are contracting in a consistent pattern over a period of time, such as walking or cycling. This kind of activity helps you relax and let your mind wander. If you do this regularly, it can be a very powerful stress reducer and can decrease symptoms of depression and anxiety.

The idea is to be completely focused on an activity or exercise to the point where you seem to have no thoughts at all. You disappear into the motion. You aren't thinking about anything. You are just there. As a result of being fully "in" your experience, you not only optimize the physical elements of the activity, you practise habits of mindfulness, ideation, and relaxation.

Movement can be a form of meditation and can trigger creativity and ideation. It's an incredible feeling. Meditative moving is also something that was natural for us as children. I have this great picture of

1% TIP: USE MOVEMENT TO SPARK YOUR BRAIN

Give your brain energy by engaging your body in a steady stream of short bursts of activity throughout the day. Think of it as microdosing—on exercise, not hallucinogens! You will find it makes a huge difference to your attention, focus, and execution. Try adding this sequence to your day:

7:00 a.m.	Morning run
8:30 a.m.	Walk to coffee shop
9:30 a.m.	20 squats ·
11:00 a.m.	10 push-ups
12:00 p.m.	15-minute walk during lunchtime
2:00 p.m.	5 minutes of stretching: hip openers, calf raises, shoulder rolls
3:30 p.m.	Plank pose (hold for 30 seconds and progress to 2 minutes, as you are able)
5:00 p.m.	Transition ritual: Find a space on the way home where you can chill for a few minutes and/or go for a walk to burn off stress from the day

my son, Adam, at age one and a half. We were on a beach in Maine, and he just wandered off on his own. I let him go because I could tell he was deep into his experience, and I knew he was totally safe. The ease of his movement, the calm in his eyes . . . it was amazing. I think it's how we should all try to be whenever we move.

Adam was doing something that came naturally to him, and I hope this sparks you to consider adding some mindful movement to your life as well. If you need a little more inspiration, consider this: Charles Darwin built a path near his home where he could walk and think while moving. President Harry Truman would start his day with a 1.5- to 3-kilometre vigorous walk. Charles Dickens would go for long walks, often at night, to help him decompress from long hours spent writing.

You can think of it as either movement practice or moving meditation—just try to avoid calling it a "workout" (see page 69). Adopting the meditative practice mindset can be very powerful.

Whether you engage in aerobic activity on its own or combined with meditation, you will improve your physical health and mental performance dramatically. You will also learn to enter into a state of relaxation that will boost your creative capacity more easily. It's a win-win-win situation.

A simple movement protocol to help you relax and boost creativity
Here are some examples of how you can train yourself in moving meditation. If you are out for a run, ride, or walk, check in with yourself to see what's happening with your thoughts and in your body. If your mind is all over the place or you feel awful and the effort is a real struggle, stop and take a break. Find a comfortable place to sit down and put yourself through

a simple 5-minute meditation. Just sit and give your complete attention to your body. Feel and count your breaths. Focus on releasing tension from specific parts of your body. Think about energy flowing into your arms, legs, chest, brain. Then, once you have brought your attention into the moment, get up and go again. When you do, I'm guessing you will experience increased ease of movement accompanied by an improvement in performance—just because you stopped to reconnect your mind and body.

Another way to practise mindful movement is to perform particular activities with 100% awareness of the motion. For example, try walking barefoot through grass. Which muscles are firing and when? How is your foot hitting the ground? What is happening with your upper body? Can you feel the blood and electricity flowing through you? How's your posture? Where is your head in relation to your neck? You can also do it through simple movements like standing up from a chair. Is your core engaged? Are you pushing up from the hips or hauling yourself up with your arms? Is the motion fluid? Are your muscles working together? Are you efficient? By tuning in so carefully, you build your capacity to engage not just in mindful movement but in a more mindful life where you can be completely present in all of your experiences: playing in the park with your kids, gardening, riding your bike, talking to your spouse.

If you can adopt moving meditation, you will find that it brings joy and creative energy to your life in ways you never considered. Here are some tips to get you started:

1. **Give yourself at least 15 minutes.** Give yourself a break and the time you need to move until your mind slows down and relaxes. The first time you go out, you might even notice that your mind becomes more active. That's okay. After a few sessions, you'll be able to relax your mind while moving your body.

2. **Go easy.** You don't want to be exercising so hard that it's uncomfortable. This type of exercise should be light. A good way to tell if you're exercising at the right intensity is that you should be breathing more quickly than when you're sitting down—just enough so you can hear air moving in and out of your nose and mouth, but not so much more that conversation would be difficult.

3. **Use music, not TV.** Listening to music while you move is okay as long as it puts you in a relaxed state. I'd recommend choosing one album or playlist that helps you relax. Don't put it on shuffle: You could be listening to a nice classical piece and in a great place mentally, then be jolted by the opening chords of an AC/DC song. Watching TV on a treadmill or bike in the gym also defeats the purpose. Just put on the headphones and allow yourself to move and let your mind wander.

It's not difficult to add some stress-relieving movement to your day. Choose a rhythmic activity you like, take it outside, take it easy, and listen to some relaxing music. This physical activity will do a lot of good for your mental state and will help you calm your mind and open up your potential to ideate, solve problems, and be creative.

1% TIP: LOSE YOURSELF IN THE MOMENT

For optimal performance, practise achieving the state of being where you are completely lost in the moment. Learn to move into a state where your brain is functioning fully and you are making connections with your potential. Bring your attention into the moment. If you are walking, think about how your feet feel when they touch the ground and how your muscles feel as they propel you forward. If you are listening to music, really listen. If you are with someone, give them 100% of your attention.

THE TAKEAWAY ON DOING LESS AND CREATIVE THINKING

We are living through one of the greatest revolutions in human history. Microprocessors have given us the internet, mobile phones, and, more recently, artificial intelligence (AI). AI has the potential to dramatically influence and disrupt the workplace in the coming years. Self-driving cars are the obvious next disruptive technology, but AI will also impact law, banking, medicine, and other industries. With the advent of AI, creative thinking becomes ever more critical.

The stream of breakthrough ideas that will make the world a better place relies on us developing novel strategies, techniques, and experiences that leverage new technologies. As Bob Moritz, the chairman of the professional services firm PwC, was quoted recently at the World Economic Forum's annual summit in Davos,

Switzerland: "We're still looking for creativity, because that can't be coded. Robotics and computers and coding actually give you a very straight and narrow path to go down a fine course. The world we're living in today is a lot more zigzag, and people are going to be important to that equation."

The issue of creativity versus productivity can be very confusing. There *is* a difference between what you need to do to be creative and what you need to do to be productive. I think they're very different things.

I've only started to figure this out based on some work that I did in the mountains of India, where I took my family to explore meditation and mindfulness and attention. I discovered that if you're 100% attentive to the moment, with no thoughts other than what exists in that moment, you've found the pure state of existence. It is so easy to be joyful when you are in that state: It's where you can access happiness, it's where you can access deep thinking, it's where you can access your true potential as a human being. I actually think it's the resting state for humanity.

Open yourself up to those *aha!* moments that can change the course of a life. Go further, higher, deeper—bring newness into your life. As you continue to learn how to relax and tap into your creativity, make sure you find ways to feed and continually improve your projects and ideas. I hope this book is helping you do this.

STEP 5: EMBRACE THE EXTRAORDINARY

"It is not the critic who counts; not the man who points out how the strong man stumbles, or where the doer of deeds could have done them better. The credit belongs to the man who is actually in the arena, whose face is marred by dust and sweat and blood; who strives valiantly; who errs, who comes short again and again; who at the best knows in the end the triumph of high achievement, and who at the worst, if he fails, at least fails while daring greatly, so that his place shall never be with those cold and timid souls who neither know victory nor defeat."
—THEODORE ROOSEVELT

I followed the steps of the climber in front of me. Between laboured breaths, a pounding heart, fuzzy vision, headache, burning muscles, pinpricks of snow burning the exposed skin on my face, and the constant presence of fear, we worked our way up Ecuador's Chimborazo volcano in the middle of the night.

I've done a lot of crazy-difficult expeditions in my life. Chimborazo was the hardest I have ever worked, physically, mentally, and emotionally. As a volcano, it gradually gets more challenging because the higher you go, the steeper it gets—and the more ice, snow, and rock you need to navigate. As the terrain gets more trying and dangerous, there is less oxygen in the air and you move more slowly. Then fatigue sets in, and the mental war gets fierce. Layer on top of that the stress associated with the falling rocks around you, the 55-degree slope, the darkness of night, a 900-metre cliff beside you, and a family back home that relies on you, and fear becomes another player in your mind–body battle.

But we continued to work our way up the mountain through the night.

It stopped snowing and got darker. We had broken through the clouds and the sky opened up overhead. I stopped climbing and raised my eyes up from the ground, over my friends in front of me, and toward the sky. "Hey, everyone, look up," I said. The line stopped, silence descended, heads lifted, and someone said, "Holy shit."

You see, we weren't just farther from the earth's centre than we had ever been: We were also the closest humans on the planet to the stars. That's why we were there. That was our dream, our drive, our vow, our commitment. We were operating at the peak of our physical and mental capacity for this very reason. We wanted to touch the sky.

I saw more stars than I thought a sky could hold. My sense of awe and wonder made the risk, pain, fatigue, and fear all worth it. I'll remember that moment for the rest of my life. It's imprinted on me, like a tattoo.

Then the lead guide put his head down and resumed climbing. We all followed, and the suffering continued.

Ultimately, my colleagues Gillian White and Sara Thompson, along with their guide, made it all the way to the summit. The rest of us got to about 6,000 metres, having reached our absolute limits, and made the decision to return to the camp safely.

Despite how hard it was, I know every person on that expedition would say it was the experience of a lifetime and that they would do it again in an instant. I'm also sure that the sight of our galaxy laid out above us is burned into their consciousness, too. That expedition gave us the opportunity to live life to the absolute limits of our human potential.

We all have ferocious potential, and it's more possible to realize this potential than many of us believe. In this chapter, we'll look at the science and practice behind optimal human performance and health, to explore how we reach our potential—whether for a single moment, a few hours, or longer.

1% TIP: PRACTISE STOP

The next time you feel suffocated by the pressure of a situation, practise STOP: Stop, Take a breath, Observe, and Proceed. Here are the four steps:

1. Stop whatever you're doing and become aware of the present moment.
2. Take a breath. Or two. Or ten.
3. Observe your body. Scan it for any sensations, tension, and emotions that are present.
4. Proceed. Carry on with life and set an intention guided by "What's most important as I move forward?" It may even be that you need to cycle through STOP again.

This tactic helps you bring your awareness into the moment so you can respond to the challenges you are faced with in the best possible way.

PIVOT FROM ROUTINE TO EXTRAORDINARY

Remember my story about swimming with sharks? On one afternoon during that vacation, Judith and I were snorkelling above a reef. I was wearing huge fins and goggles. As we were swimming, we noticed that the reef had dropped off below us. All we could see were fish. Judith tapped my side. I looked back and she motioned to the right. There was a 6-foot reef shark swimming up beside me.

By now you know that I used to be a competitive swimmer. So what do I do when another swimmer gets close to me? I race.

I sped up. I could see the shark's dorsal fin over the water alongside me. *I was swimming with the shark right next to me.* In that brief moment, I could see the shark's eye. I could see its teeth. I could see the pores on its skin. I could see the way it was moving. I could see the individual muscles along its body. I could tap my feet in sync with the rhythm of its fin strokes.

It was one of the coolest 30 seconds of my life. And during that brief experience, though I didn't have an fMRI strapped on me to prove it, I am certain my brain was firing gamma brainwaves (created in moments of peak experience, synchrony, and connection). It was a moment of peak experience. Everything was possible. My entire history as a swimmer, my environmental awareness, my background as an exercise scientist, my connection to the ocean— everything was firing.

You don't necessarily need to swim with sharks to get into a gamma state and experience life at a different level. You can actually learn to activate this state of all-in performance. You can trigger gamma brainwaves and that moment of synchrony when everything comes together. You can learn to enter a state where your brain is functioning fully and you are making connections with your true potential in that moment.

I've talked about movement and meditation, both of which train people to get into peak states more often. Now I'm going to share how to enter and sustain your zone. Along with that comes experiencing joy, music, gratitude, and connections to the great people around you. All of these factors can increase your ability to control your mental and physical health so you can engage deeply with what matters the most to you and experience all that life has to offer.

Extraordinary moments begin with getting into the flow and opening up to peak experience.

Get into the Flow

Have you ever been completely focused and absorbed in your exercise only to emerge an hour later and realize you just did some of your best training? Or were able to perform at a level you never knew you were capable of until that moment? A moment in which your mind quieted down and you effortlessly flowed through the steps?

Just about everyone can identify with experiences like these. Unfortunately, for most of us, these moments are rare and seem random. But when we explore the science of human performance, you'll see that this zone—also known as *flow*—is something you can achieve; it is a state you can control.

Flow was first described by Mihaly Csikszentmihalyi, who identified it as a highly focused state conducive to peak performance and productivity. Being in "the zone" or a "flow" state is

155

characterized by complete absorption in an activity and being entirely in the present (no sense of past or future). You feel a loss of time—hours have gone by but it seems like only moments.

In the research literature, the "ideal performance state" (also known as "the zone") was first described by psychologists Robert M. Yerkes and John Dillingham Dodson in 1908. When our activation is too low, we lack motivation, interest, and energy. When our activation is too high, we are agitated, anxious, stressed, or tense. When we are in flow, which I think is an extension and deepening of being "in the zone," we become so engrossed in the activity that the world seems to fade away. Nothing else seems to matter. There is *automaticity* (action without the need for deliberate attention upon execution) in the performance and no internal judgment.

Somewhere between these two activation states (not enough and too much) lies the ideal performance state where we are most likely to enter the transcendent state known as flow. Flow is when we are energized, motivated, focused, happy, and able to perform at our best. Csikszentmihalyi describes eight characteristics of flow: concentration on the task, clarity of goals, transformation of time, intrinsic reward, effortlessness, a balance of challenge and skills, a merging of actions and awareness, and a feeling of control.

Your ideal state for a given task depends on the task. When I'm playing with my daughter, I have to be almost meditative, slow and calm. Before public speaking, I have to get really psyched up. I activate my body just like I used to before a swim race. I try to get a bit nervous so I have great energy to start the talk. For television appearances, I have to have energy and clarity of thought and total focus. If I'm thinking about anything other than the topic of the day, the appearance does not go well.

The ideal performance state exists between the two extremes of low and high activation. Knowing what you need—and how to ignite your body and mind to prepare for that demand—can help you build your own peak performance zone. You can learn how to access your most productive mode in every area of your life.

To begin, you need to practise removing all distractions, worries, and unnecessary mental activities from your mind—this is the mode where you disappear, where you fully immerse yourself in the moment and the activity. Once you have done it a few times, you will know how it feels and what you need to do to make it happen. Then you'll be able to replicate it and enter the zone on demand.

Whether applied to an athletic activity or when sitting at your desk, practice and repetition will help you get your body and mind into the zone—neither too relaxed nor too wired—so you can achieve your goals more easily.

If you follow these steps, you can develop a deliberate process for fully immersing yourself in any activity you wish.

Before you begin, remove yourself from all distractions and unnecessary mental activities.

1. **Identify your best zone moment.** Think of a time when you achieved something great and were in a particularly good zone. Find the right language (or even images) to describe the moment to yourself. Single words can be helpful: Maybe they include where you were, what you were doing, and how you felt. Using pictures as a reference is okay, too. Visualize anything that reminds you of the actions, thoughts, and feelings that happened during your optimal performance.

2. **Remember what it felt like.** Now try to recall exactly what you were doing (body), thinking (mind), and feeling (emotions) before and during your flow performance. Write down any additional words that specifically describe each.

3. **Build your zone routine.** Identify three things that you can do to recreate your iconic past performances in the future. What physical resources do you need (a particular space and any support materials)? What thoughts and actions will move you closer to the state you described above? The key is to build a picture of your ideal performance state so you can trigger that state by acting like you did when you were in it. From there, the thoughts and feelings will follow. If you get distracted or tension slips in, take control. Make some changes. Breathe your way into it. Move differently, think differently, transition to a different emotional state.

Once you have practised deliberately entering your zone a few times, it will become easier to replicate the experience. As they say, practise makes progress.

1% TIP: BREATHE YOUR WAY INTO THE ZONE

Breathing is effective because the centres of your brain that control breathing are closely linked to the area that controls stress. If you can calm the electrical activity in the breathing centre, then you have a good chance of calming the stress. Deep, controlled breathing to calm anxiety or stress is often called *combat breathing*. You can do it anytime you feel that you are slipping out of your zone or having trouble getting into it.

OPEN UP TO PEAK EXPERIENCE

We can probably all identify with a flow state moment. The run where everything felt easy, the day at work where you got loads done and time seemed to fly by, the moment of joy with your kids. Peak experience has most of the same characteristics as flow, with one key difference: Peak experience moments are transformative in that they have a meaning that changes your perspective on life.

As I was writing this chapter, I messaged Dr. Gillian White, who was completing her Ph.D. at the time. I asked her, "If you were to describe the Chimborazo experience in one word, how would you describe it?" She cheated and said, "recalibrated perspective." Then she carried on with "deep internal reflection" and "real f'ing awesome." It was an intense challenge that created the opportunity for awe in the moment. It was so powerful that it made us all adjust how we thought about and experienced life long after the event happened.

While most people can identify with a moment of flow, fewer people report having experienced peak experience. Peak experiences are states where we have peak performance along with full clarity of self in the process. Gayle Privette, a researcher at the University of West Florida, suggests that peak experience involves "a heightened sense of wonder, awe, or ecstasy over an experience." An example that many people can relate to is falling deeply in love with someone, but peak experiences can happen in sports, music, the arts, nature, and during many other pursuits.

Generally, there appear to be three core characteristics of peak experiences:

1. A sense of significance that leads to an increase in personal awareness or understanding;
2. A sense of fulfillment where the experience generates positive emotions and is intrinsically rewarding; and
3. A sense of connection and losing track of time.

These moments of peak experience may occur privately, perhaps as a moment of sudden insight while writing. They may occur in public, perhaps during a speech when you are in the zone or while listening to or performing music at a concert. But whatever it is and whoever else sees or experiences it, its meaning is deeply personal.

Gord Downie of the Tragically Hip was the national poet of Canada for over 30 years. He was always an intensely personal man who kept himself, as a person, out of the public eye. After he was diagnosed with terminal brain cancer, he did something uncharacteristic: He shared his personal news with the world. Then he and the Hip released one more album and went on one last tour together.

The Tragically Hip's final concert was broadcast all across Canada and around the world, and millions of people tuned in. During the concert, despite his struggle with cancer, Downie completely unleashed his love, energy, creativity, and passion. He was raw and open and there for the audience and his art all the way through. Knowing he had the attention of the entire country during one of the encores, he spoke at length about Truth and Reconciliation, the history of First Nations peoples in Canada, and the residential school system characterized by cultural assimilation and attempted genocide. And as he talked, he spoke directly to

1% TIP: CONSIDER YOUR IMPACT

Be aware of the impact that your successes will have. This impact can be on you, your family, your teammates, your clients, your students, the country, or even the world. I have decided that my professional mission is to help 1 billion people be healthier and reach their potential. In my family life, my sole focus is on empowering my children as they grow into their lives.

Being clear about the potential impact of your team and your own work is a huge motivator. More importantly, it can make people content despite the challenges that often accompany trying to make a difference in the world. Knowing you will have an impact will also keep you going when obstacles and setbacks abound.

What impact do you seek to have in the world? Write it down and share it at every opportunity.

Prime Minister Justin Trudeau and challenged him to lead the way and make it right.

I believe that the potential impact of those comments, that moment, was one of the main reasons Downie made a commitment to that final tour. When he came offstage, you could see on his face how much finishing his life as a musician in this particular way mattered to him. He was dying, but he had purpose and meaning. His body was giving out, but he was operating at a level well beyond the ordinary, even for a live concert situation.

Downie's story illustrates the power of personal meaning. His impact on others was and still is profound. But his concert, his address to the prime minister, and his work to raise awareness of historical wrongs and abuses committed against Canada's

Indigenous peoples came from a deeply personal place. As a musi-cian, he happened to have a public venue. But as a person, he was focused on a truth and a purpose that came from deep inside. He did something that mattered to him. It was a moment of ultra-performance within a caring and compassionate life.

So, what is that for you?

PEAK EXPERIENCE, EXTRAORDINARY MOMENTS, AND GAMMA BRAINWAVES

As interest in brainwaves as measured by EEG has increased and expanded, researchers have discovered gamma waves (see page 19). Gamma waves are fast, high-frequency, rhythmic brain responses that have been shown to spike when higher cognitive processes are engaged. This knowledge is so new that there is still some debate about the existence of these waves and their relevance. But there is enough evidence to share the idea with you, even if only to illustrate what gamma waves represent: a state of being where ultra-performance is possible.

Gamma waves appear to originate in the base of your brain, in the visual cortex, and sweep forward across your brain at a rate of between 30 and 100 cycles per second (Hz). Gamma states are influenced by sensory input (sight, sound, feel, taste, touch) and processes in the brain including working memory, perception, and attention. Gamma states occur when you are in the moment, taking in information about your environment, processing that information against your established memories and experiences, all while your attention is in the here and now.

Gamma waves are evident during a peak state. This is what elite performers achieve: a gamma state of ultra-performance. Think Alex Honnold free climbing El Capitan, Usain Bolt warming up and racing, Neil Armstrong and Buzz Aldrin landing on the moon, or Marie Curie working in her lab and making a key discovery. Even better, think about yourself: sitting on a stunningly beautiful beach at sunset, completely present in the moment; or staring deeply into the eyes of a loved one; or holding your child for the first time. While we may not be exactly in gamma in each of these moments, we are in states of peak human potential and performance, where everything comes together and we ascend to a new level in our lives.

In this state, things happen in the body and brain that we are only just beginning to understand.

Interestingly, gamma waves have been measured both in people in deep meditation and in people actively engaged in moments of pure extraordinary experience: That bike ride when you forget you're cycling. That speech when you were so dominant you lost track of yourself. That moment with your partner when you're completely locked in on each other. That instant when you see the shape of your sculpture emerge or your experiment succeed or your presentation win the room. These are all gamma wave moments, when various brain networks engage all at once and we have peak perception and function.

Gamma is when you are operating at the limit of your capacity and nothing is getting in your way. It's when you can embrace the extraordinary.

THE KEYS TO EXPERIENCING AND EMBRACING THE EXTRAORDINARY

Your Chimborazo climb can be any moment of personal meaningful achievement. It's something that takes time and effort to reach and create, but when you're there, it feels like everything in you is fully engaged and firing at once. It's a moment that draws on your passion and talent. You feel an internal sense of accomplishment. You're not in it for anyone else, though others may be lightly or even profoundly affected. You are connected to your own purpose and are fully yourself.

So what is that? Where do you want to go? What do you want to do? What stands majestically ahead of you, like a rock face that inspires awe and gets your blood flowing just thinking about it?

You and I might not be the world's greatest musician—or athlete, scientist, artist, or entrepreneur—but we share something in common with all of them: We can learn to achieve a state of ultra-performance that enables us to reach the limit of our own abilities.

We know we need to ditch our fear of failure to get there: to stop seeing failure as a referendum on our worth and instead view it as useful feedback for greater growth. We know we need to be fuelled by internal motivation and personal meaning, not praise or awards, or we'll give up when we falter. In addition, I believe that positive mental habits and experiences act as jet packs that launch us toward exceptional performance. *It's not how fast you swim, it's how you swim fast.*

The elements along the journey to high performance need to be positive, even pleasurable, for you to achieve your best. The four keys below will bring delight and joy to the "how you swim fast" part of your personal ultra-performance.

Key #1 (Brain): Pivot from External Validation to Intrinsic Motivation

If your sense of success or failure comes from outside of you—whether through accepting the judgment of others or through internalizing that judgment and using it against yourself—then so does your sense of accomplishment. If you feel your happiest or most satisfied when you receive external validation and rewards, then your sense of who you are and how good of a person you are comes from others. That's a dangerous way to live.

Fearing external judgment and relying on external validation to feel good are equally problematic. And both are a barrier to achieving high performance.

Far away from fear and the need for external validation (praise, admiration, awards, approval) lies meaning. Terminally ill patients never wish they had been praised and admired more. They don't wish they had earned more employee-of-the-month plaques. They are focused on internal questions of meaning: being true to themselves, having closer relationships, wishing work hadn't defined them so much. They don't think so much about the *what* of life—their jobs or material possessions or trophies—but on the *why* of life. *It's not what you do, but why you do it.* It's not the individual task or challenge, but the significance of your choices or actions.

What matters to us is an important question, because one thing we have learned about meaning and motivation is that when we are driven to perform from deep within ourselves, we do our best work and we feel good about it. When we are driven to perform from outside ourselves, for praise and rewards, our motivation falls off and we don't do as well. We've got the wrong *why*.

Here's a story to illustrate how powerful personal meaning and knowing our *why* can be. When we think of Michael Phelps, the first thing that comes to mind is that he has won more Olympic medals than any other athlete in history. What many people don't realize is that despite, or perhaps as a side effect of, all of his money, fame, and success, Phelps went through what many of us experience in our careers and lives: a dark period. When training was a grind, Phelps fell into darkness. When it was a joy, he reached new heights.

In 2014, halfway between Olympic Games, Phelps was deeply depressed and really struggling in every area of his life. At one point he was photographed smoking weed out of a bong and was twice charged with driving under the influence, including once in a school zone. At his lowest point, he called his coach, explained that he was having thoughts about suicide, and said, "I've had it. I can't take this anymore." The coach helped Phelps get into rehab.

While in rehab, Phelps wasn't one of the most successful athletes in history. He was just a guy working through the steps. One of them was making calls to friends and family to make amends. Reconnect with people. Talk through what had happened. Work it through—for himself and for them.

When he was on a call with his best friend, the conversation didn't unfold as Phelps had expected. The friend challenged him by asking a simple question that ended up changing the course of Phelps's life: "Is that the best that you can do?" Reflecting on the question, Phelps realized that what had happened so far, though amazing by any external standard, wasn't even close to all he was capable of and wanted to achieve. Stepping back, he realized that he had been focusing on the *what* (the medals), not the *why* (his passion for training, pushing limits, giving his best, and loving the sport). Phelps left rehab soon after and returned to his training with a new focus on enjoying and embracing the process. He changed his diet. He committed to physical therapy. He added yoga, stretching, massage, and functional training to his swimming. He repaired a number of relationships. And, maybe most important of all, he stopped reading magazines and started reading biographies of people like Mahatma Gandhi and Steve Jobs—role models of meaning and purpose.

Fast-forward to 2016 and the Rio Olympics: Phelps was a picture of happiness. During all of the media interviews he gave, his themes were being there to try his hardest, to not end up with regret, and to know that he had left it all out there in the lanes.

By pivoting his thinking from external validation and awards to his own meaning and values, Phelps re-energized his life and rediscovered his purpose. He let go of fear. He let go of judgment. He put feelings of failure aside. And then he lived the life he loved. *That's* the power of internal motivation and meaning. And it lies at the heart of optimization and high performance. Your peak moments need to be driven by something much deeper than praise or trophies: They must be fuelled by meaning, by your personal sense of value and purpose. External rewards are fine in the right mindset and can be fun to have once in a while. But they are not the meaning of our lives and they will not sustain us in our pursuit of excellence in the long term.

A simple protocol to help eliminate the fear of failure

The antithesis of being in the zone, in a flow state, in gamma, is also the enemy of ultra-performance: negative emotion. Anger, fear, resentment, regret, jealousy. When we let those emotions into our hearts and into our lives, they destroy our ability to perform.

In 2009, Australian Bronnie Ware was a budding author and songwriter. She also happened to have spent close to a decade working as a palliative care nurse. That year, she wrote a blog post reporting on things that her terminally ill patients wished they had done differently. The post went viral, changing her life and leading to her international bestseller, *Top Five Regrets of the Dying*.

When Ware interviewed people on their deathbeds, they shared regrets like "I wish I had the courage to live a life that was true to myself," "I wish I had spent more time with friends and family," "I wish I had expressed my true feelings more," "I wish I hadn't worked so hard," and "I wish I'd pursued happiness."

The regrets of these terminally ill patients offer us an important opportunity to shift our perspective on failure.

People who have achieved immense success invariably say that before they got it right, they got it colossally wrong. Many times. And they will point out that they were able to capitalize on those failures because they saw them as a gift, not a curse. Elite athletes don't get to the top of their sport by having competed against people they could beat. They pushed themselves to the limit so that they failed—again and again. Then they used the information and experience from those setbacks to get better.

Or consider relationships. Every strong bond I know of, whether professional or personal, got that way with the help of some kind of conflict, misunderstanding, and tension. Colliding with each other and then sorting out what happened is an essential part of solidifying a partnership.

Somehow, we have to get rid of our underlying belief that failure is embarrassing, a sign of weakness, or an indication that we are not cut out to succeed. To think differently, we have to embrace—deeply and fully—the idea that there is no way to achieve your potential if you don't put yourself in situations where you will fail, and then do it with gusto. Maybe not happily, but with passion and determination.

We have to reframe failure as an essential ingredient in growth. By perceiving it as a challenge rather than a threat, we can amplify our lives.

In particular, I think leaders, coaches, teachers, and parents have to change the failure narrative. It's up to us to create an environment where our employees, players, students, and children feel safe. They need to know we will not hammer them if they falter. That not only is it okay to leap and fall short, it is the only way to go. Otherwise, they will always be paralyzed by negative thinking about their ability.

I also think that everyone in a position of influence needs to model positive responses to failure. Don't cover up your miscues. Don't act like all is well. Be up front and honest when you get it right and when you get it wrong. Show everyone who relies on you that setbacks and less-than-ideal performances are embraced. Show them how to grow. Show yourself how to grow.

Build Your Personal Positive Community
In his book *The Blue Zones of Happiness: Lessons from the World's Happiest People*, which looks at regions around the world where

people seem to have a high chance of living to become centenarians, Dan Buettner suggests that one of the keys to longevity is consistent social connection: "The people we surround ourselves with, even friends of friends, strongly influence our health. We create connections in a community—between individuals and community organizations, faith-based and community groups, and other social activities—so you can easily connect with your right tribe. As we say, belong to live long."

Your personal environment is not insignificant. Your brain is flexible, constantly under construction, and you respond greatly to your surroundings and your habits. You can empower or dampen your potential depending on your environment. The best thing about this is that you get to decide who you want to be by creating the conditions around you.

It has been said that we are the sum of the five people we spend the most time with. This applies to the amount of money we make, our fitness level, and our happiness. Which leads to an important question about the people around you: Are they making you better? Whatever you are trying to accomplish, make sure you surround yourself with people who elevate you and who you can elevate in turn.

But what makes a terrific community? Is it putting the greatest minds together? Socializing outside of work? Grouping people by experience? Having the same level of education? Having a strong leader?

Positive communities might have some or all of those things. But so do groups that have problems. No doubt you know what a poorly functional, not-so-productive "team" is like. People report feeling pretty low, doubtful of their own ability, sometimes even emotionally damaged when they've been part of a low-functioning or failing team. On the other hand, a really great team delivers a boost of energy and confidence that lasts beyond the time you spend together.

Don't confuse a bad team with a really tough situation or problem to solve. On one of the best teams I ever formed, we all experienced freezing conditions, physically gruelling 18-hour days, and rough working conditions (as in setting up an "office" on the side of a cliff using solar panels to run a satellite network). You recognize the place: We were 6,000 metres up in the Andes on Chimborazo. We were often cold, hungry, tired, sometimes even sick . . . and happy. And we were successful. The living was hard, but the teamwork was fantastic. We were on a high when we got back from the expedition. Our team members had quite a few things in common, including some fancy credentials and unusual expertise. But that wasn't why we worked. It's not enough to have "the best people." There's much more to a great team than that.

How much more? That's what Google asked itself about 5 years ago when it embarked on Project Aristotle. Google studied hundreds of its own teams and discovered this: How a team functions is far more important than who is on it. The team's "communal health" matters the most. It's not about how smart the members are; it's about how they view their task and treat one another.

So when you put together a team, you actually don't need the brainiest people, or the people with the most academic degrees or business certificates, or the people at higher levels of accomplishment than you. Don't get me wrong. Any of those folks might be great—so long as their view of the task and their commitment to a positive collaboration matches yours. Look for people with the right mindset: passionate, engaged, positive, supportive of others.

These are the people who will help carry you to high performance (while you also carry them).

Key #2 (Body): Get Fit, Fast, Strong, and Flexible

Physical activity can dramatically improve your health and performance. If you want to live a world-class life, you'll need an exercise plan. In particular, you'll want an approach that capitalizes on what I call the 4 Fs: Fit, Fast, Force (aka Strong), and Flexible.

Get Fit

By "Fit," I mean cardiovascular endurance. I want your heart, lungs, blood, and circulatory vessels to be healthy and high functioning. Each time you walk, jog, run, swim, or bike, and you sustain that exercise for longer than 20 minutes, you trigger a number of positive adaptations in the body. Your heart muscles get stronger and the chambers in your heart increase in size so they can pump more blood. You get more alveoli (microscopic air sacs where oxygen and carbon dioxide are exchanged between the air and the lungs). Cardiovascular exercise also increases the number of capillaries in your muscles and organs. All of these adaptations come together over time to help you feel energetic, prevent you from getting sick, and give you the opportunity to reach your potential at anything you're passionate about. Try doing some sort of cardiovascular aerobic endurance—an activity that raises your heart rate and makes you sweat—three times a week. People usually think of running, but there are lots of options: Go for a walk. Go for a bike ride. Get out on a paddleboard. It doesn't matter. Just raise your heart rate and sweat. Research has proven that this is an essential way to extend your life.

Get Fast

"Fast" simply means moving quickly, and interval training (alternating between going fast and taking it easier, as in a spin class or when resting between sets) is a great way to make that happen. Interval training can improve both your endurance capacity (aerobic energy system and type I muscles) and your strength capacity (anaerobic energy system and type II muscles). When you do that, you teach your body how to process metabolic waste more efficiently, which improves your overall fitness and increases your ability to recover on the fly. Once in a while, skip your strength training and do something fast instead, an all-out activity that builds up the lactic acid in your muscles and causes that "feel the burn" sensation. You can do it any way you want. Just slide in a spin class or sprint session when you would normally lift weights, and then knock yourself out.

Get Strong

It is so important that you train your muscles to create more force, which helps you become stronger. Exercise science tells us that when you do strength training (also known as resistance training), you are engaging a different energy system and muscle fibres than you use when you're doing cardiovascular endurance training. As long as you maintain a reasonable intensity, strength training will require the kind of force that is generated by your type II muscle fibres (your speed and strength muscle fibres) and your anaerobic energy system (the twin engines that get involved when you sprint, jump, or do heavy lifting). Do some sort of strength training twice a week. This one is important as we age, especially for maintaining our bone and muscle mass. By strength training, you can amplify your performance and stimulate the growth of neurons in your brain.

Get Flexible

I'd like you to spend some time each week (ideally a little bit every afternoon or evening) stretching. Stretching calms you down by activating your parasympathetic nervous system (the recovery and regeneration system). Even if you have had a brutal day, as I sometimes do working in the cancer ward at SickKids, coming home and doing 20 minutes of stretching or yoga makes a huge difference. And if you want to sleep like you haven't slept in years, do three or four restful yoga poses, take a hot bath followed by a cold shower, meditate for 10 minutes, read some fiction, and turn out the light.

That's it. Other than that, I suggest doing something active and fun on Sundays, and also taking one day a week off to recover and regenerate. Even world-class athletes take a break once a week. Use the 4 Fs to optimize your health and performance so you feel great all the time.

WORDS OF WISDOM: ALEX HUTCHINSON ON THE POWER OF EXERCISING WITH A GROUP

Alex Hutchinson is an author, scientist, and journalist who writes for Outside *magazine,* Running World, *and* The Globe and Mail. *Alex has a Ph.D. in physics from the University of Cambridge and competed as a middle- and long-distance runner for the Canadian national team.*

One area that I find most interesting is the literature in evolutionary anthropology on social bonding, the origins of collective behaviour, and how and why we work together. One of the classic examples is a study conducted with the rowing team at Oxford. We know that pain tolerance increases from endorphins released during exercise. So they compared the increase when rowers trained on their own versus what happened when they trained with the entire team. The increase in pain tolerance was about twice as big when the group trained together. There was something about performing the task in the presence of teammates that produced a bigger change in brain chemistry.

Key #3 (Space): Manifest the Power of Gratitude

In the past two decades, researchers have learned that gratitude is strongly related to all aspects of well-being. Gratitude has even been shown to reduce mental-health disorders such as depression, anxiety, and post-traumatic stress disorder (PTSD). A person who has suffered a traumatic experience, for example, is able to recover better and even achieve a higher level of emotional well-being afterward if they are oriented toward noticing and appreciating the positive in the world.

Adopting a "gratitude attitude" reduces stress, lowers heart rate, decreases inflammation in the body, improves sleep, strengthens relationships, reduces conflict, and triggers reciprocally helpful behaviour. This last finding means that a person who shows gratitude—for a friend's input, a home-cooked meal, a parent's help with homework—increases the likelihood that the recipient of the gratitude will show more care and compassion toward others. Gratitude generates kind-hearted acts (referred to in the scientific literature as "prosociality") like the ripples of a pebble dropped in water.

Let's start with understanding the component parts of gratitude:

- **An appreciation of other people:** "I'm lucky to have David as a friend/teammate/brother."
- **A focus on what you currently have:** "I'm thankful for my family/for the healthy food available/for a safe and warm home."
- **Feelings of awe when encountering beauty:** "This waterfall is a wonder!"
- **Focusing on the positive in the present moment:** "I'm going to sit here on this park bench for a moment and take in the autumn colours."
- **Feelings of gratitude arising from the understanding that life is short:** "I will die and people I know will die, so this day matters so much."
- **Positive social comparisons:** "There are so many people who have less than I do."

Considering this list, you can see that gratitude is not naive, immature, or disconnected from reality. In fact, it's mostly generated from the very real, sometimes even serious, features of our lives.

Key #4 (Practice): Use Music to Enhance Your Life

If you think about how music affects us—from pumping us up to filling us with pleasure or bringing tears to our eyes—it's not hard to recognize that music, especially live music, has a powerful effect on the brain and body.

Music can help energize your body, activate your brain, reduce fatigue, and increase your performance. For example, if we listen to music while exercising, our bodies pick up on the pace and flow of the music and start to mirror it. Music can even make a tough workout feel easier to complete. Studies show that endurance is increased when listening to music and that motivational music—whatever personally lights you up—has an impact on stamina.

Along with changing your mood and energy, music can also have an important effect on your brain's ability to execute. Listening to or studying music consistently remodels your brain and enables you to function at a higher level. MRI scans have shown that the pathways in your brain affected by music run from the cochlea in your ear through the auditory nerve and into the basal centres of your brain (the very, very early centres of the brain that run up into and through your limbic system, the emotional centre of your brain). This means that listening to or playing music amplifies your brain— which means you can use music to amplify your life.

Stefan Koelsch, professor of music psychology at the University of Berlin, published a literature review that documents the effects of music on individuals and groups, and identified the following "seven Cs" of music. Music provides opportunities for:

1. Social **contact** with other human beings;
2. Dramatic increases in **cognition** (the function of your brain);
3. **Co-pathy** (empathy shared with others);
4. **Communication** (sharing lyrics and experiences);

5. More effective **coordination** (people are attuned to each other);
6. Enhanced **cooperation** (because of shared experience); and
7. Greater **cohesion** among groups.

Throughout time, music has been an important and universal part of society. It can have a powerful effect on our emotions and mood. We are just starting to learn about the interactions between music as a performance enhancer and as a way for us to improve our mental health.

Because music affects the limbic system, a region of our brain associated with emotions, if we create a soundtrack for our lives, we can use music to help us get excited, energized, and focused, or, on the other hand, relaxed, calm, and joyful. Align your music with your life and amazing things can happen. Oh yeah—and get a good set of headphones!

A simple protocol to help you leverage the power of music
Use music on your way to work to get ready for whatever lies ahead. Use music to transition to new activities, like the deep concentration required for a project or at the end of the day when you need to wind down.

Make a handful of playlists that help for a variety of situations. If you're feeling tense and anxious and don't even want to get moving at all, listen to a calming soundtrack—songs that touch you personally and engage your emotions in a soothing manner—to lower your heart rate and de-stress. You can also use a calming soundtrack when walking or practising moving meditation (see page 143) or even doing household chores.

Create as many soundtracks for your life as you like. Put music to work for you.

THE TAKEAWAY ON EXTRAORDINARY EXPERIENCES

Remember when I told you about climbing the volcano in the middle of the night and seeing the stars? Well, that successful summit almost didn't happen.

Just a few days before, my team was training on the mountain when suddenly the temperature dropped, clouds blocked the sun, and the atmospheric pressure fell. As a result, we all developed altitude sickness. We decided to get off the mountain as quickly as possible.

Descending a mountain while nauseated and dizzy, and with a blinding headache, is not easy or fun. I measured my blood oxygen saturation at 66%. When healthy humans are at rest at sea level, blood oxygen levels are expected to be at 99% to 100%. When athletes are in competition, their levels can drop as low as 85%. People who are having lung or heart problems may also experience low levels, and any value below 85% usually triggers a visit to the emergency room. So, to put it mildly, we were having a hard time.

A few hours later, we were all safely back at our lodge at the base of the mountain to rest and recover. As physiologists, we measure ourselves constantly, and we had brought equipment with us to track our health and performance. Over the next few days, we noticed interesting changes in our bodies after that brutal experience: They started to adapt. We built new red blood cells, and our hemoglobin levels jumped. Our muscles healed and we felt stronger. Our VO_2 max (a technical term for maximal aerobic capacity, or maximum endurance capacity) increased, which meant that our entire oxygen transport system (responsible for taking oxygen out of the air and transferring it into our muscles and brain) improved dramatically.

The physical, mental, and emotional struggle we experienced in low oxygen just a few days before had stimulated our bodies and brains to change for the better—and fast. And that adaptation happened while we were resting *after* the training climb. We trained hard, we rested, and then we got better.

A few days later, when we attempted the summit for the last time, our bodies were able to handle the atmospheric pressure changes, the cold, the physical strain of climbing up ice, and the mental stress of pushing ourselves to the limit. All of this set the stage for the extraordinary experience of being the closest humans to the stars!

By doing less, we accomplished more. We experienced the limits of what life has to offer when we paused to see the universe unfold above our heads. At its most fundamental, that is what this book is about. I hope that I have helped you slow down so you can experience all the wonder, joy, and awe in your life.

TIME SHIFT:
SIMPLE WAYS TO RECHARGE, WHETHER YOU HAVE SECONDS, MINUTES, AN HOUR, A DAY, A WEEK, OR MORE

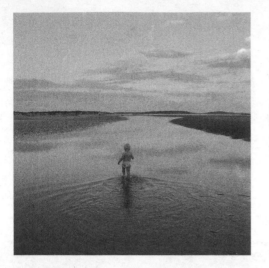
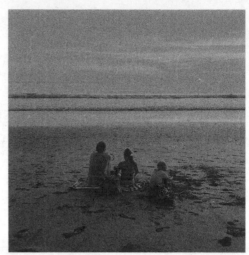
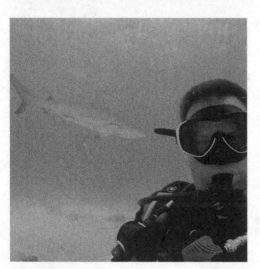
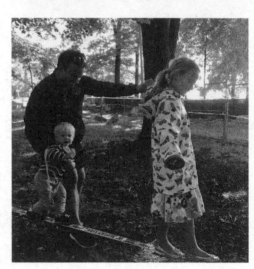
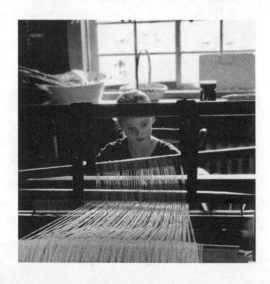
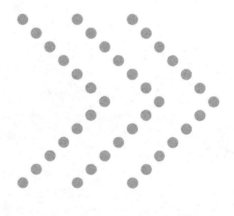

My dream with this book is to help you slow down so you can recover, regenerate, and recharge your body, mind, and life. I want you to be healthy, to do what you love at the highest level possible, and to reach your ultimate potential. I want you to feel better, to have more energy, to be able to think clearly, to learn, to create, to be happy, to overcome obstacles, to crush challenges, and to dominate your competition.

When you put these strategies into practice, you can start to craft your life deliberately rather than simply reacting to the stream of constant demands coming at you. You can take control. You can be intentional. You can focus and grow. You can make the most of what life brings you in each moment. You won't be perfect—that's just life and that's fine. But you can start to move the needle toward a healthy, happy life that you'll be able to look back on with contentment.

This chapter presents a framework for practically applying the ideas in this book no matter how much time you have: 1 second, 1 minute, 1 hour, 1 day, 1 week, or 1 month. I hope this gives you some ideas about how you can implement the principles in this book. One suggestion might resonate with you more than others, and that's okay—go with it.

I HAVE SECONDS TO RECHARGE

Okay, you're about to blow up. You're stressed. You're tired. You've just had it. You want to respond, not react. What do you do? Here are some ways you can press the pause button, if even for only a few seconds.

Idea 1: Do a big stretch

Remember that the enemies of performance and health are tension and fatigue. Stretching your muscles will help you dissipate tension and feel better, even if you just do one big stretch. While lying down, sitting, or standing, extend your body as long as you can, from your toes to the top of your head, and reach up to the sky. Then you can . . .

Idea 2: Take a deep breath

Taking a few seconds to breathe slowly and deeply can change your physiology for the better. It can help calm you down if you are stressed and energize you with life-giving oxygen if you're tired. Breathe in deeply, then slowly exhale. Repeat a few times. Then re-engage with whatever is going on around you.

Idea 3: Drink some water

Water is the fundamental nutrient your body needs to create energy. Pausing to take a drink of water can give you a few seconds to disconnect from what you are currently doing and give your body what it needs to get healthy and perform better. (If you want to dig deeper into the benefits of hydration, I cover it in more detail in my previous book *The Ripple Effect*.)

Idea 4: Remember what is important

Sometimes a little dose of perspective can work wonders. Ask yourself, "Will this moment matter in an hour, a day, a month, or a year?" Of course, some things are legitimately important, but often we'll get worked up over what seems like a big issue in the moment when, if we paused to really consider what matters, we'd realize we can take the pressure off ourselves.

Idea 5: Do a body scan

Take a breath, sit or stand up straight, and bring your attention to your body. Beginning at your head and working down, scan your body and release tension each time you exhale. Relax your face, shoulders, chest, back, stomach, arms, legs, hands, and feet. The more you practise this, the faster you'll be able to do it.

Ultimately the goal here is to create some time and space between stimulus and response so you can act with response-ability, rather than simply reacting compulsively.

I HAVE MINUTES TO RECHARGE

Imagine you are a musician, minutes before your performance starts—the crowd is energized and you're about to go out there and do your thing. Or you might be a student who has just sat down in an exam hall to write a key exam. Or a businessperson about to deliver a key presentation. Or an athlete stepping up to the starting blocks. How do you ensure that you're ready and in the zone?

Idea 1: Get in the zone and Act-Think-Feel

The key here is making sure that you are not too far at either end of the spectrum: too stressed or tense or too relaxed or tired. If you need to calm down, take a few deep breaths, focus on the process not the outcome (that is, technique not medals), and use the Act–Think–Feel approach from Step 4 (see 124) to get activated and energized.

Idea 2: Be mindful

Bringing your attention into the here and now, where it belongs, is a powerful tool for controlling your body, mind, and emotions so you can focus on what you need to do (and as little else as possible) at the highest level in the moments that matter. Great athletes make their sports look effortless because they have refined their technique to eliminate everything not critical to the performance. Mindfulness can help you achieve that mindset in just a few minutes.

Idea 3: Get cold

You may not be able to jump into a cold shower to spark your adrenaline response, but it's something I highly recommend if you can swing it. On big performance days, finishing your morning shower with a few minutes of cold water can help sharpen your mind. Another strategy is to get some fresh air. I do this every chance I get before speaking engagements.

Idea 4: Listen to one song

Taking a short break to put on some headphones and listen to a great piece of music can be a game changer—that's why you often see Olympic athletes listening to music right up until the moment they step up to race. Use your favourite tune to psych you up or calm you down, depending on what you need in the moment.

Idea 5: Practise gratitude

Need to reset your mindset? Take a few minutes to jot down the five things you are most grateful for in your life right now. Doing this simple practice will help you focus on what is important so you can avoid getting caught up in short-term issues.

What we are looking to do in just a few minutes is to get ourselves into our ideal performance state, a positive place in which we are energized and can do our best.

I HAVE AN HOUR TO RECHARGE

The ability to put space and time between a stressor or challenge and your actions and responses can be key to success in so many situations. With a whole hour to commit to ourselves, we can change our mindset, physiology, and performance so we can refuel, improve our fitness, and really set ourselves up for sustainable excellence.

Idea 1: Get in a workout

If you have an hour, why not practise? Take a yoga or spin class, lift some weights, or go for a walk or run. Get your blood flowing, increase your body temperature, and release some brain-derived neurotrophic factor (BDNF) to recharge your brain and body. A little exercise can also help dissipate stress hormones and reset your emotions. Remember that you don't need the whole hour: You'll reap benefits with as little as 15 minutes.

Idea 2: Take a nap

The research is clear: 20-minute power naps can help improve concentration, alertness, and focus. Longer naps of 75 to 90 minutes are great for mental and physical recharging. Just avoid taking 45- to 60-minute naps, when it's more likely you'll wake up out of deep sleep with sleep inertia. So grab a pillow—the power of a nap is undeniable.

Idea 3: Meditate, walk, refuel

Taking a break to meditate will give your brain a rest and restore you mentally, physically, and emotionally. I love 20 minutes of meditation to clear and settle my mind. If you can, follow your meditation with a 20-minute power walk. It's a powerful combination to spark creativity and problem-solving. The final piece of this micropractice is to take 20 minutes to eat a healthy power snack. I call this my middle-of-the-day 20–20–20 protocol.

Idea 4: Take a sauna

If you have access to a sauna, give yourself an hour to get hot. Get into the heat and stay until you're sweating, then get out and take a cool to cold shower. Repeat two or three times. Finish with a cool shower until you stop sweating. Dry off, drink cool water to rehydrate, and take 10 minutes to notice how deeply relaxed you feel.

Idea 5: Be absolutely alone

Sometimes we just need to be by ourselves, with no distractions. Go for a walk in the park and leave your phone behind. I love swimming because no one can call me in the pool. Go to your local coffee shop with some headphones and a great book. Take some time with yourself.

With an hour we can take a real break to dissipate stress, rest, re-energize, refuel, and set the stage for better health and unlocking true human potential.

I HAVE A DAY TO RECHARGE

When we have days at our disposal, we have all sorts of options for really regenerating, not just recovering. When we give ourselves more time, we can help the body and brain actually change. Energy is created, muscles are rebuilt, and neurons are grown.

Idea 1: Get a good sleep

When you get a good sleep—that's 7 to 8 hours—then your brain and body heal, recover, and regenerate optimally. You'll encode memories and set yourself up for maximum creativity. Your muscles will repair and your nervous system will optimize. It all starts with sleep.

Idea 2: Skip a meal

While this might be counterintuitive, giving yourself a break from eating and digesting can help speed physiological regeneration. When we skip a meal, either breakfast or dinner, we activate the benefits of intermittent fasting (see page 37). You'll be surprised how quickly the hunger passes and how good you feel the next morning.

Idea 3: Give yourself some time to really think

We rarely have enough time to really plan things out. Strategic thinking and planning are so important to making sure our lives are headed in the right direction. Take some time and get into metacognition by asking three questions: what, why, and how.

Idea 4: Get into nature

Have a day off? Perhaps there's some nice weather forecasted for this weekend. Why not go to a park or the beach? Go for a bike ride or a paddle. Eat with friends or family outdoors. Being in nature improves our physical and mental health. Get out there. Along the same lines, I have found that visiting art galleries and museums has a similar effect. It's not nature, but it does change my mindset for the better.

Idea 5: Reconnect

Once in a while I love to take a day to deliberately reconnect with family and friends. I'll scroll through my address book and send messages to people I have not seen or talked to recently. This usually sparks some phone calls, direct messages, and online chats with people. I love my community and try to keep building it up so I can keep in touch with the people who matter to me the most.

With a day we can truly recharge and begin to access greater energy, creativity, ideation, and peak experiences.

I HAVE A WEEK (OR MORE) TO RECHARGE

Alright. Here we are near the end of the book. You're inspired. You're a believer. You're ready to take the next big step and join the real Recharge Revolution. The game changer is to take a whole week off, or maybe even 2 or 3 weeks in a row, to rest, recover, reset, refocus, regenerate, and recharge.

Idea 1: Take a real vacation

Plan a great getaway with family or friends, or even just by yourself. Find somewhere that inspires and heals. Discover the world the places where you can get better. I've had the great pleasure of travelling to over 50 countries. I've done trips by myself, with friends, with teams as an athlete and coach, with business colleagues, with family, and alone with my wife. I don't regret a single trip. They were all different, and they all made me and my life better in some way. Trips don't have to be major expeditions. They can be to a nearby national park for some camping. They can be staycations where you disconnect and spend some time relaxing at home with your family. Or you can ski to the South Pole by yourself, like my buddy Ray Zahab. Your call.

Idea 2: Do some deep inner work

On page 85 I wrote about intrinsic versus extrinsic motivation. It is worth taking the time to figure out what really drives you. I needed time—a lot of time—to sit and think about what I really wanted to do in my life before it became clear (at least for the moment). To kickstart yourself, check out my podcast with Philip McKernan at **http://bit.ly/PhilipMcKernanPodcast**.

Idea 3: Read a book

Pick up a great biography or brilliant work of fiction. Find an author or topic that informs or inspires you. Great books give you the chance to have a conversation with the author or learn an entirely new idea or topic. Build your library. I encourage the CEOs that I coach to read a new book at least every 2 weeks.

Idea 4: Learn something new

We live in a world with nearly unlimited access to information and training. When we take some time to be creative and learn, new opportunities and experiences emerge. I had a friend who took a week to learn how to forge swords. Others have gone on silent meditation retreats. My athlete friends will go to a training camp to practise new sports skills. Anything counts. This is all about process, not outcome. It may not even matter what you are learning or creating, just that you're trying something new.

When we take a week or even a month to deliberately recharge, we set ourselves up to be able to perform at the highest level possible in a sustainable way. Alternating between high-performance and deep recovery is what can bring balance and health to our lives.

I sincerely hope these ideas help you put the concepts from this book into practice in your own life.

With infinite gratitude—
Greg Wells

ACKNOWLEDGEMENTS

Everything begins and ends with my family. Judith, Ingrid, and Adam, I have missed you (again) while writing this book. Your patience, love, and support are the best, and I am so lucky that you are who I get to spend life with. Judith is the Greatest. Wife. Ever.

I've had every opportunity in this wonderful life, and a huge part of that is because of my incredible parents. Mom and Dad, thanks so much for everything you do for all of us.

My fantastic extended family showers me with love and support, and everything is great as a result. Sarah, Brent, Sadie, Declan, Margaret, David, Benedict, Thompson, Terry, and Chris, thanks so much for making life so special for all of us.

In my work life, I get to spend time at one of the most amazing institutions in the world: the Hospital for Sick Children in Toronto, Canada. There I am surrounded by some of the most intelligent, thoughtful, and supportive professionals anywhere. Every day that I get to do research at SickKids is a good day. Thanks for helping me think, learn, and create better.

I'd also like to thank my lab team, who are so fun, smart, hard-working, and dedicated. The world will be so much better off thanks to all of you and all that you do. The team at Wells Performance are equally brilliant, and we are going to change the world together. Thank you, all.

In this book I've cited hundreds of articles, studies, and books. Many of the ideas that I have shared here come from people who have joined me on my podcast. I have also travelled extensively, speaking at conferences, and I have seen the best of the best on various stages at transformative events all over the world. I have learned so much from so many people. I am once again standing on the shoulders of giants. I am so grateful.

My practice as a performance physiologist has placed me with some of the best performers on the planet in many different disciplines. These people have enabled me to help them reach their potential. There is really nothing I love doing more than helping others get better at whatever they do. To all the athletes, patients, business professionals, students, teachers, principals, pilots, musicians, and military personnel that I have had the opportunity to spend time with—thank you for trusting me and giving me the chance to work with you.

Near the end of writing this book, I had a few blocks and struggles. One day I sent a text message to a dozen friends asking a key question about human potential. My friends are busy and have many obligations. They are some wildly accomplished, supremely cool, loving humans. But despite how much they have going on, within 1 hour, all 12 had responded to me with thoughts and ideas that were insightful and powerful. The point is that, when I needed them, every single one came through. I think I might have the best groups of close friends anyone could ever ask for.

Finally, thanks to my world-class editor, Brad Wilson, and the HarperCollins team. I'm quite sure I was a difficult author to get through the publishing process this time, and I appreciate you all. I'm thankful to have the opportunity to publish my fourth book with you.

NOTES

STEP 1: RECOVER DELIBERATELY

9   *Meanwhile, according to the Nielsen Total Audience Report for 2019*: The Nielsen Company. "The Total Audience Report: Q1 2016" (2016). Available at www.nielsen.com/us/en/insights/report/2016/the-total -audience-report-q1-2016/.

10   *Sleep deprivation isn't pretty. According to the Centers for Disease Control (CDC)*: Centers for Disease Control & Prevention (CDC). "Unhealthy sleep-related behaviors—12 states" (2011). *Morbidity and Mortality Weekly Report* 60, no. 8: 233–38.

10   *A study by Dr. Judith Ricci*: Ricci, J.A., E. Chee, A.L. Lorandeau, and J. Berger. "Fatigue in the US workforce: Prevalence and implications for lost productive work time." *Journal of Occupational and Environmental Medicine* 49, no. 1 (February 2007): 1–10.

10   *Scientists in Finland have determined that burnout and exhaustion*: Toppinen-Tanner, S., A. Ojajärvi, A. Väänänen, R. Kalimo, and P. Jäppinen. "Burnout

as a predictor of medically certified sick-leave absences and their diagnosed causes." *Behavioral Medicine* (Washington, DC) 31, no. 1 (Spring 2005): 18–27.

10   *associated with a decline in three main cognitive functions: executive functions, attention, and memory*: Deligkaris, P., E. Panagopoulou, A.J. Montgomery, and E. Masoura. "Job burnout and cognitive functioning: A systematic review." *Work & Stress: An International Journal of Work, Health & Organisations* 28, no. 2 (2014): 107–23.

14   *exercising clarity appears to change a structure in the brain called the* inferior frontal cortex: Hampshire, A., S.R. Chamberlain, M.M. Monti, J. Duncan, and A.M. Owen. "The role of the right inferior frontal gyrus: Inhibition and attentional control." *Neuroimage* 50, no. 3 (April 15, 2010): 1313–19; Chong, T.T., M.A. Williams, R. Cunnington, and J.B. Mattingley. "Selective attention modulates inferior frontal gyrus activity during action observation." *Neuroimage* 40, no. 1 (March 1, 2008): 298–307.

14   *Bruce Bowser, founder and chair of AMJ Campbell, tells people that when he gets on an airplane he can bang out 30 or 40 emails very quickly*: Personal communication with Dr. Greg Wells.

15   *Her first Harry Potter manuscript was rejected by 12 publishers*: Oswald, A. "Even rockstar author JK Rowling has received letters of rejection." *Insider* (July 28, 2016). Available at www.insider.com/jk-rowlings-rejection-letters-2016-7.

16   *Beth Ford, CEO of Land O'Lakes, was quoted in* Fast Company *magazine*: Ford, B., as told to C. Weissman. "Land O'Lakes CEO Beth Ford has one rule about email." *Fast Company* (November 27, 2018). Available at www.fastcompany.com/90263519/land-olakes-ceo-beth-ford-has-one-rule-about-email.

17   *When I interviewed Alex Hutchinson*: Episode 3 of *The Dr. Greg Wells Podcast.* "Alex Hutchinson on the Limits of Human Performance" (September 11, 2018). Available at https://anchor.fm/dr-greg-wells/episodes/3--Alex-Hutchinson-on-the-Limits-of-Human-Performance-e1rjrg.

18   *Words of Wisdom: Judith Humphrey*: Episode 14 of *The Dr. Greg Wells Podcast.* "Judith Humphrey on Leading through Communication" (December 4, 2018). Available at https://anchor.fm/dr-greg-wells/episodes/14--Judith-Humphrey-on-Leading-through-Communication-e1rjqt.

21   *20% of Americans have a diagnosed sleep disorder*: Maternal and Child Health Bureau. "Sleep disorders." *Women's Health USA 2011* (2011). Available at https://mchb.hrsa.gov/whusa11/hstat/hshi/pages/224sd.html.

21   *1 in 10 people suffer from chronic insomnia*: Cleveland Clinic. "Insomnia" (2018). Available at https://my.clevelandclinic.org/health/diseases/12119-insomnia.

21   *97% of teenagers get less than the recommended amount of sleep each night*:
Winsler, A., A. Deutsch, R.D. Vorona, P.A. Payne, and M. Szklo-Coxe.
"Sleepless in Fairfax: The difference one more hour of sleep can make for
teen hopelessness, suicidal ideation, and substance use." *Journal of Youth
and Adolescence* 44, no. 2 (February 2015): 362–78.

21   *comes increased rates of obesity, heart attack, stroke, cancer, depression, and
anxiety*: Centers for Disease Control and Prevention. "Short sleep duration among US adults" (Last reviewed May 2, 2017). Available at www
.cdc.gov/sleep/data_statistics.html.

21   *over 1 million people . . . reported that sleeping less than 6 hours a night was
associated with increased mortality*: Mazzotti, D.R., C. Guindalini, W.A.
Moraes, M.L. Andersen, M.S. Cendoroglo, L.R. Ramos, and S. Tufik.
"Human longevity is associated with regular sleep patterns, maintenance
of slow-wave sleep, and favorable lipid profile." *Frontiers in Aging Neuroscience* 6 (June 24, 2014): 134.

21   *sleep deprivation, which the Centers for Disease Control defines as 6 or fewer
hours per night*: Centers for Disease Control and Prevention. "Short sleep
duration among US adults" (Last reviewed May 2, 2017). Available at
www.cdc.gov/sleep/data_statistics.html.

22   *Dr. Hiraku Takeuchi and colleagues . . . performed brain imaging*: Takeuchi, H., Y. Taki, R. Nouchi, R. Yokoyama, Y. Kotozaki, S. Nakagawa,
A. Sekiguchi, K. Iizuka, Y. Yamamoto, S. Hanawa, et al. "Shorter sleep
duration and better sleep quality are associated with greater tissue density
in the brain." *Scientific Reports* 8, no. 1 (April 11, 2018): 5833.

22   *the prefrontal cortex, where higher-level thinking occurs and dopaminergic
systems of the brain . . . are located*: Luo, S.X., and E.J. Huang. "Dopaminergic neurons and brain reward pathways: From neurogenesis to
circuit assembly." *American Journal of Pathology* 186, no. 3 (March 2016):
478–88.

22   *the primary role of sleep is regulating the repair, regeneration, and optimization of the nervous system*: Mourrain, P. "What lies sleeping: Why can
science still not define this most basic biological process?" *The Scientist*
(Thought Experiment) (March 1, 2016).

23   *NREM sleep seems to be when we establish new connections between neurons
in the brain*: Maquet, P. "The role of sleep in learning and memory." *Science* (New York, NY) 294, no. 5544 (November 2, 2001): 1048–52.

23   *Dr. Dierdre Barrett from the Department of Psychiatry at Harvard Medical
School argues*: Harvard Catalyst. "Deirdre Leigh Barrett, Ph.D.: Over-
view." *Harvard Catalyst Profiles*. Available at https://connects.catalyst
.harvard.edu/Profiles/display/Person/39720.

23   *Stage 1 of NREM sleep is related to mental flexibility*: Drago, V., P.S. Fos-
          ter, K.M. Heilman, D. Aricò, J. Williamson, P. Montagna, and R. Ferri.
          "Cyclic alternating pattern in sleep and its relationship to creativity." *Sleep
          Medicine* 12, no. 4 (April 2011): 361–66.

23–24   *the natural cyclical pattern of sleep . . . is important for originality and diver-
          gent thinking*: Drago, V., P.S. Foster, K.M. Heilman, D. Aricò, J. William-
          son, P. Montagna, and R. Ferri. "Cyclic alternating pattern in sleep and its
          relationship to creativity." *Sleep Medicine* 12, no. 4 (April 2011): 361–66.

24   *interesting research on the link between sleep and learning*: Tamminen, J.,
          R.M.A. Lambon, and P.A. Lewis. "The role of sleep spindles and slow-
          wave activity in integrating new information in semantic memory." *Jour-
          nal of Neuroscience* 33, no. 39 (September 2013): 15376–81.

24   *exercise has beneficial effects on total sleep time*: Kredlow, M.A., M.C.
          Capozzoli, B.A. Hearon, A.W. Calkins, and M.W. Otto. "The effects of
          physical activity on sleep: A meta-analytic review." *Journal of Behavioral
          Medicine* 38, no. 3 (June 2015): 427–49.

25   *Professor Michael Scullin and colleagues . . . did a different experiment*: Scul-
          lin, M., M. McDaniel, D. Howard, and C. Kudelka. "Sleep and testing
          promote conceptual learning of classroom materials." Presented at the
          25th Anniversary Meeting of the Associated Professional Sleep Societies
          LLC, Minneapolis, MN (June 2011).

25   *strengthens your immune system, helping to keep colds, flu bugs, inflamma-
          tion, and infection at bay*: Besedovsky, L., T. Lange, and J. Born. "Sleep
          and immune function." *Pflugers Archive* 463, no. 1 (January 2012): 121–37.

31   *regular stretching can relieve muscle tension, reduce pain, and improve range
          of motion*: Garber, C.E., B. Blissmer, M.R. Deschenes, B.A. Franklin, M.J.
          Lamonte, I.M. Lee, D.C. Nieman, and D.P. Swain. "Quantity and quality
          of exercise for developing and maintaining cardiorespiratory, musculo-
          skeletal, and neuromotor fitness in apparently healthy adults: Guidance
          for prescribing exercise." American College of Sports Medicine Posi-
          tion Stand. *Medicine & Science in Sports & Exercise* 43, no. 7 (July 2011):
          1334–59.

31   *when activities like sitting compromise our health, stretching can be a huge
          help*: Alter, M.J., *Science of Flexibility*, 3rd ed. Champaign, IL: Human
          Kinetics Publications, 2004.

31   *static stretching increasing the activity of the parasympathetic (rest and recover)
          nervous system*: Saito, T., T. Hono, and M. Miyachi. "Effects of stretching
          on cerebrocortical and autonomic nervous system activities and systemic
          circulation." *American Journal of Physical Medicine & Rehabilitation* 12
          (2001): 2–9.

32   *sympathetic nervous system activity, along with heart rate and blood pressure, increased*: Takayuki, I., T. Shimizu, R. Baba, and A. Nakagaki. "Acute changes in autonomic nerve activity during passive static stretching." *American Journal of Sports Science and Medicine* 2, no. 4 (2014): 166–70.

32   *Similar findings have been shown for people who practise yoga*: Khattab, K., A.A. Khattab, J. Ortak, G. Richardt, and H. Bonnemeier. "Iyengar yoga increases cardiac parasympathetic nervous modulation among healthy yoga practitioners." *Evidence-Based Complementary Alternative Medicine*, no. 4 (2007): 511–17.

32   *Similar findings have been shown for people who practise . . . Tai Chi*: Lu, W.A., and C.D. Kuo. "The effect of Tai Chi Chu'an on the autonomic nervous modulation in older persons." *Medicine & Science in Sports & Exercise* 35, no. 12 (December 2003): 1972–76.

34   *obesity damages muscle tissue, which in turn causes exercise intolerance*: Wells, G.D., L. Bank, J.E. Caterini, S. Thompson, M.D. Noseworthy, T. Rayner, C. Syme, B.W. McCrindle, and J. Hamilton. "The association among skeletal muscle phosphocreatine recovery, adiposity, and insulin resistance in children." *Pediatric Obesity* 12, no. 2 (April 2017): 163–70.

37   *to help prevent or treat cardiovascular disease, diabetes, cancer, obesity, and dementia*: Longo, V.D., and S. Panda. "Fasting, circadian rhythms, and time-restricted feeding in healthy lifespan." *Cell Metabolism* 23, no. 6 (June 14, 2016): 1048–59.

37   *evidence for the benefits of intermittent fasting is compelling*: Di Francesco, A., C. Di Germanio, M. Bernier, and R. de Cabo. "A time to fast." *Science* 362, no. 6416 (November 16, 2018): 770–75.

37   *has been shown to improve longevity in animal models*: Speakman, J.R., and S.E. Mitchell. "Caloric restriction." *Molecular Aspects of Medicine* 32, no. 3 (June 2011): 159–221.

37   *Calorie-restricted eating has been shown to increase the incidence of disordered eating and anorexia*: Walford, R.L., D. Mock, R. Verdery, and T. MacCallum. "Calorie restriction in biosphere 2: Alterations in physiologic, hematologic, hormonal, and biochemical parameters in humans restricted for a 2-year period." *Journals of Gerontology: Series A, Biological Sciences and Medical Sciences* 57, no. 6 (June 2002): B211–24.

38   *followed by eating normally on the other days*: Longo, V.D., and S. Panda. "Fasting, circadian rhythms, and time-restricted feeding in healthy lifespan." *Cell Metabolism* 23, no. 6 (June 14, 2016): 1048–59.

38   *protect against obesity, cardiovascular disease, hypertension, diabetes, and neurodegenerative diseases*: Mattson, M.P., D.B. Allison, L. Fontana, M.

Harvie, V.D. Longo, W.J. Malaisse, M. Mosley, L. Notterpek, E. Ravussin, F.A. Scheer, et al. "Meal frequency and timing in health and disease." *Proceedings of the National Academy of Sciences of the United States of America* 111, no. 47 (November 25, 2014): 16647–53.

38   *as well as slow the growth of tumours*: Varady, K.A., S. Bhutani, E.C. Church, and M.C. Klempel. "Short-term modified alternate-day fasting: A novel dietary strategy for weight loss and cardioprotection in obese adults." *American Journal of Clinical Nutrition* 90 (November 12, 2009): 1138–43.

38   *Human studies have been promising in terms of weight loss and cardiometabolic health*: Carlson, O., B. Martin, K.S. Stote, E. Golden, S. Maudsley, S.S. Najjar, L. Ferrucci, D.K. Ingram, D.L. Longo, W.V. Rumpler, et al. "Impact of reduced meal frequency without caloric restriction on glucose regulation in healthy, normal-weight middle-aged men and women." *Metabolism: Clinical and Experimental* 56 (2007): 1729–34.

38   *improved lipid profiles, lower blood pressure, and increased insulin sensitivity*: Lee, C., L. Raffaghello, S. Brandhorst, F.M. Safdie, G. Bianchi, A. Martin-Montalvo, V. Pistoia, M. Wei, S. Hwang, A. Merlino, et al. "Fasting cycles retard growth of tumors and sensitize a range of cancer cell types to chemotherapy." *Science Translation Medicine* 4, no. 124 (March 7, 2012): 124ra27.

38   *a fascinating study on time-restricted feeding (fasting) during Ramadan*: Cherif, A., B. Roelands, R. Meeusen, and K. Chamari. "Effects of intermittent fasting, caloric restriction, and Ramadan intermittent fasting on cognitive performance at rest and during exercise in adults." *Sports Medicine* (Auckland, New Zealand) 46, no. 1 (January 2016): 35–47.

39   *can delay the onset and progression of diseases and lead to a healthier, longer life*: Di Francesco, A., C. Di Germanio, M. Bernier, and R. de Cabo. "A time to fast." *Science* 362, no. 6416 (November 16, 2018): 770–75.

39   *A related impact of time-restricted feeding is that it increases* autophagy: VerPlank, J.J.S., S. Lokireddy, J. Zhao, and A.L. Goldberg. "26S proteasomes are rapidly activated by diverse hormones and physiological states that raise cAMP and cause Rpn6 phosphorylation." *Proceedings of the National Academy of Sciences of the United States of America* 116, no. 10 (March 5, 2019): 4228–37; first published February 19, 2019.

39   *Pairing time-restricted feeding with exercise appears to enhance this process in humans*: Pesheva, E., HMS Communications. "Exercise, fasting help cells shed defective proteins." *The Harvard Gazette: Health & Medicine.* (February 21, 2019). Available at https://news.harvard.edu/gazette/story/2019/02/exercise-fasting-shown-to-help-cells-shed-defective-proteins/.

39   *The combination of fasting and exercise also stimulates neurogenesis*: Marosi,
      K., and M.P. Mattson. "BDNF mediates adaptive brain and body
      responses to energetic challenges." *Trends in Endocrinology and Metabo-
      lism* 25, no. 2 (February 2014): 89–98.

42   *vacation use has been in a steady decline since 2000*: US Travel Association.
      "Time off and vacation usage" (2019). Available at www.ustravel.org
      /toolkit/time-and-vacation-usage.

43   *Changing work culture can also have a profound positive impact*: Denis, K.
      "Emailing while you're on vacation is a quick way to ruin company cul-
      ture." *Harvard Business Review* (December 5, 2017). Available at https://
      hbr.org/2017/12/emailing-while-youre-on-vacation-is-a-quick-way-to
      -ruin-company-culture.

43–44 *being in work mode all the time exhausts the focus circuits in the brain, which
      drains mental energy and reduces self-control*: Pillay, S. "Your brain can only
      take so much focus." *Harvard Business Review* (May 12, 2017). Available
      at https://hbr.org/2017/05/your-brain-can-only-take-so-much-focus.

44   *time away from work improves well-being*: de Bloom, J., M. Kompier, S.
      Geurts, C. de Weerth, T. Taris, and S.J. Sonnentag. "Do we recover from
      vacation? Meta-analysis of vacation effects on health and well-being."
      Journal of Occupational Health 51, no. 1 (2009): 13–25.

44   *time away from work . . . reduces the risk of metabolic syndrome*: Hruska, B.,
      S.D. Pressman, K. Bendinskas, and B.B. Gump. "Vacation frequency is
      associated with metabolic syndrome and symptoms." *Psychological and
      Health* 17 (June 2019): 1–15.

44   *time away from work . . . improves heart health*: Neumayr, G., and P.
      Lechleitner. "Effects of a one-week vacation with various activity pro-
      grams on cardiovascular parameters." *Journal of Sports Medicine and Phys-
      ical Fitness* 59, no. 2 (February 2019): 335–39.

44   *time away from work . . . might even be protective against depression*: Kim,
      D. "Does paid vacation leave protect against depression among working
      Americans? A national longitudinal fixed effects analysis." *Scandinavian
      Journal of Work, Environment and Health* 45, no. 1 (January 1, 2019): 22–32.

44   *a shorter, less immersive vacation has been shown to improve health and
      well-being*: de Bloom, J., S.A. Geurts, and M.A. Kompier. "Effects of
      short vacations, vacation activities and experiences on employee health
      and well-being." *Stress Health: Journal for the International Society for the
      Investigation of Stress* 28, no. 4 (October 2012): 305–18.

44   *a shorter, less immersive vacation . . . can even improve cardiovascular health
      parameters*: Neumayr, G., and P. Lechleitner. "Effects of a one-week
      vacation with various activity programs on cardiovascular parameters."

Journal of Sports Medicine and Physical Fitness 59, no. 2 (February 2019): 335–39.

44   *as soon as you get home from your holiday you start planning the next one*: de Bloom, J., M. Kompier, S. Geurts, C. de Weerth, T. Taris, and S. Sonnentag. "Do we recover from vacation? Meta-analysis of vacation effects on health and well-being." *Journal of Occupational Health* 51, no. 1 (2009): 13–25.

46   *being in natural settings improves health and reduces stress*: Hartig, T., R. Mitchell, S. de Vries, and H. Frumkin. "Nature and health." *Annual Review of Public Health* 35 (2014): 207–28.

STEP 2: THINK ABOUT HOW YOU THINK

50   *chronic stress contributes to high blood pressure, promotes the formation of artery-clogging deposits, and causes brain changes that contribute to anxiety, depression, and addiction*: Harvard Health Publications, Harvard Medical School. "Understanding the stress response: Chronic activation of this survival mechanism impairs health." Available at https://nowcomment .com/documents/78537.

51   *American Psychological Association's 2010 Stress in America Survey*: American Psychological Association. "APA survey raises concern about health impact of stress on children and families" (November 9, 2010). Available at www.apa.org/news/press/releases/2010/11/stress-in-america.aspx.

54   *"Between stimulus and response there is a space . . . our growth and our freedom"*: May, R. "Freedom and responsibility re-examined." In Lloyd-Jones, E., and E.M. Westervelt (eds.). *Behavioral Science and Guidance: Proposals and Perspectives*. New York: Bureau of Publications, Teachers College, Columbia University, 1963: 95.

58   *Words of Wisdom: Kunal Gupta*: Episode 16 of *The Dr. Greg Wells Podcast*. "Kunal Gupta on Finding Mindfulness in the Workplace and in Life" (December 18, 2018). Available at https://anchor.fm/dr-greg-wells /episodes/16--Kunal-Gupta-on-Finding-Mindfulness-in-the-Workplace -and-in-Life-e28bp9.

62   *Metacognition is a fascinating process that was defined by John Flavell in 1979*: Flavell, J.H. "Metacognition and cognitive monitoring: A new era of cognitive-development inquiry." *American Psychologist* 34, no. 10 (1979): 906–11.

62   *your ability to reflect and consider tasks that you have undertaken*: Saylor Academy. "What is metacognition?" Available at https://saylordotorg

.github.io/text_leading-with-cultural-intelligence/s06-02-what-is
-metacognition.html.

62   *metacognition helps students improve their grades*: Chen, P., O. Chavez, D.C. Ong, and B. Gunderson. "Strategic resource use for learning: A self-administered intervention that guides self-reflection on effective resource use enhances academic performance." *Association for Psychological Science* 28, no. 6 (June 1, 2017): 774–85.

62   *how 1,390 Ph.D. students managed their learning*: Cantwell, R.H., S.F. Bourke, J.J. Scevak, A.P. Holbrook, and J. Budd. "Doctoral candidates as learners: A study of individual differences in responses to learning and its management." *Studies in Higher Education* 42, no. 1 (May 1, 2015): 47–64.

63   *researchers have recently identified regions of the brain that are activated when we practise metacognition*: Fleming, S.M., and R.J. Dolan. "The neural basis of metacognitive ability." *Philosophical Transactions of the Royal Society of London. Series B, Biological Sciences* 367, no. 1594 (2012): 1338–49.

63   *The rostral and dorsal aspects of the prefrontal cortex appear to be very important for accuracy of retrospective analysis of performance*: Benoit, R.G., S.J. Gilbert, C.D. Frith, and P.W. Burgess. "Rostral prefrontal cortex and the focus of attention in prospective memory." *Cerebral Cortex* 22, no. 8 (August 2012): 1876–86.

64   *Ana Dutra at the Harvard Business School writes that when leaders pause and reflect*: Dutra, A. "The power of pause." *Harvard Business Review* (January 5, 2012). Available at https://hbr.org/2012/01/the-power-of-pause.

64   *research suggests that you can shift into metacognition by asking yourself three questions: what, why, and how*: Chen, P., O. Chavez, D.C. Ong, and B. Gunderson. "Strategic resource use for learning: A self-administered intervention that guides self-reflection on effective resource use enhances academic performance." *Association for Psychological Science* 28, no. 6 (June 1, 2017): 774–85.

65   *exercise stimulates the growth of new neurons*: Curlik, D.M., and T.J. Shors. "Training your brain: Do mental and physical (MAP) training enhance cognition through the process of neurogenesis in the hippocampus?" *Neuropharmacology* 64, no. 1 (2013): 506–14.

66   *12 runners were asked to perform four modes of exercise*: Brümmer, V., S. Schneider, T. Abel, T. Vogt, and H.K. Strüder. "Brain cortical activity is influenced by exercise mode and intensity." *Medicine & Science in Sports & Exercise* 43, no. 10 (2011): 1863–72.

66   *Our bodies contain a protein kinase called mTOR*: Kaeberlein, M. "mTOR inhibition: From aging to autism and beyond." Review article. Huber, O., R. Ria, and S.-Y. Shieh (eds.). *Scientifica* (Cairo, Egypt) 2013: 849186.

66   *"Broadly speaking, organisms are constantly . . . the tissue and organismal level as well"*: Kaeberlein, M. "mTOR inhibition: From aging to autism and beyond." Review article. Huber, O., R. Ria, and S.-Y. Shieh (eds.). *Scientifica* (Cairo, Egypt) 2013: 849186.

66   *extend lifespan simply by doing aerobic exercise, such as walking, jogging, cycling, or swimming*: Kaeberlein, M. "mTOR inhibition: From aging to autism and beyond." Review article. Huber, O., R. Ria, and S.-Y. Shieh (eds.). *Scientifica* (Cairo, Egypt) 2013: 849186.

66–67 *AMP kinase, an enzyme in our bodies that has a massive positive impact on everything from muscles*: Jeon, S.M. "Regulation and function of AMPK in physiology and diseases." *Experimental Molecular Medicine* 48, no. 7 (July 15, 2016): e245.

66–67 *AMP kinase . . . has massive positive impact on everything from . . . bones to the brain*: Mihaylova, M.M., and R.J. Shaw. "The AMPK signalling pathway coordinates cell growth, autophagy and metabolism." *Nature Cell Biology* 13, no. 9 (2011): 1016–23.

67   *aerobic training actually changes our DNA*: Denham, J., B.J. O'Brien, and F.J. Charchar. "Telomere length maintenance and cardiometabolic disease prevention through exercise training." *Sports Medicine* (Auckland, New Zealand) 46, no. 9 (September 2016): 1213–37; Arsenis, N.C., T. You, E.F. Ogawa, G.M. Tinsley, and L. Zuo. "Physical activity and telomere length: Impact of aging and potential mechanisms of action." *Oncotarget* 8, no. 27 (July 4, 2017): 45008–19.

67   *won Dr. Elizabeth Blackburn the Nobel Prize for Physiology and Medicine in 2009*: "Elizabeth H. Blackburn—Biographical." *The Nobel Prize* (August 29, 2019). Available at https://www.nobelprize.org/prizes/medicine/2009 /blackburn/biographical/.

67   *As we age, our telomeres shrink*: Arsenis, N.C., T. You, E.F. Ogawa, G.M. Tinsley, and L. Zuo. "Physical activity and telomere length: Impact of aging and potential mechanisms of action." *Oncotarget* 8, no. 27 (July 4, 2017): 45008–19.

67   *DNA starts to fray and come apart, which causes errors to start to accumulate*: Giardini, M.A., M. Segatto, M.S. da Silva, V.S. Nunes, and M.I. Cano. "Telomere and telomerase biology." *Progress in Molecular Biology and Translational Science* 125 (2014): 1–40.

67   *researchers compared the telomeres of runners . . . to more sedentary non-runners*: Borghini, A., G. Giardini, A. Tonacci, F. Mastorci, A. Mercuri,

S. Mrakic-Sposta, S. Moretti, M.G. Andreassi, and L. Pratali. "Chronic and acute effects of endurance training on telomere length." *Mutagenesis* 30, no. 5 (September 2015): 711–16; Rae, D.E., A. Vignaud, G.S. Butler-Browne, L.E. Thornell, C. Sinclair-Smith, E.W. Derman, M.I. Lambert, and M. Collins. "Skeletal muscle telomere length in healthy, experienced, endurance runners." *European Journal of Applied Physiology* 109, no. 2 (May 2010): 323–30.

67   *Even a 15-minute walk*: Yates, T., F. Zaccardi, N.N. Dhalwani, M.J. Davies, K. Bakrania, C.A. Celis-Morales, J.M.R. Gill, P.W. Franks, and K. Khunti. "Association of walking pace and handgrip strength with all-cause, cardiovascular, and cancer mortality: A UK Biobank observational study." *European Heart Journal* 38, no. 43 (November 14, 2017): 3232–40.

67   *Similar benefits are seen with cycling*: Celis-Morales, C.A., D.M. Lyall, P. Welsh, J. Anderson, L. Steell, Y. Guo, R. Maldonado, D.F. Mackay, J.P. Pell, N. Sattar, et al. "Association between active commuting and incident cardiovascular disease, cancer, and mortality: Prospective cohort study." *British Medical Journal* (Clinical Research Ed.) 19, no. 357 (April 2017): j1456.

68   *exercise stimulates the release of stem cells*: Emmons, R., G.M. Niemiro, O. Owolabi, and M. De Lisio. "Acute exercise mobilizes hematopoietic stem and progenitor cells and alters the mesenchymal stromal cell secretome." *Journal of Applied Physiology* (Bethesda, MD: 1985) 120, no. 6 (March 15, 2016): 624–32.

68   *change themselves into pretty much any other type of cell in the body*: Boppart, M.D., M. De Lisio, and S. Witkowski. "Exercise and stem cells." *Progress in Molecular Biology and Translational Science* 135 (2015): 423–56.

68   *the release of stem cells from our muscles and blood vessels, which then circulate around the body and repair tissue*: Emmons, R., G.M. Niemiro, O. Owolabi, and M. De Lisio. "Acute exercise mobilizes hematopoietic stem and progenitor cells and alters the mesenchymal stromal cell secretome." *Journal of Applied Physiology* (Bethesda, MD: 1985) 120, no. 6 (March 15, 2016): 624–32.

68   *positive changes in mood occur* after *physical exercise*: Schuch, F.B., D. Vancampfort, J. Richards, S. Rosenbaum, P.B. Ward, and B. Stubbs. "Exercise as a treatment for depression: A meta-analysis adjusting for publication bias." *Journal of Psychiatric Research* 77 (June 2016): 42–51.

68   *individuals who are more physically active tend to be happier in general*: Lathia, N., G.M. Sandstrom, C. Mascolo, and P.J. Rentfrow. "Happier people live more active lives: Using smartphones to link happiness and physical activity." *PLOS ONE* 12, no. 1 (2017): e0160589.

68   *higher levels of happiness ... consistent across 15 European countries*: Richards, J., X. Jiang, P. Kelly, J. Chau, A. Bauman, and D. Ding. "Don't worry, be happy: Cross-sectional associations between physical activity and happiness in 15 European countries." *BMC Public Health* 15 (2015): 53.

69   *Researchers have proven time and again that exercise boosts learning*: Davis, C.L., P.D. Tomporowski, J.E. McDowell, B.P. Austin, P.H. Miller, N.E. Yanasak, J.D. Allison, and J.A. Naglieri. "Exercise improves executive function and achievement and alters brain activation in overweight children: A randomized, controlled trial." *Health Psychology: Official Journal of the Division of Health Psychology, American Psychological Association* 30, no. 1 (January 2011): 91–98.

70   *Significant scientific evidence supports the fact that spending time in nature helps us not only relax but also get healthier*: Mygind, L., E. Kjeldsted, R.D. Hartmeyer, E. Mygind, M. Bølling, and P. Bentsen. "Immersive nature-experiences as health promotion interventions for healthy, vulnerable, and sick populations? A systematic review and appraisal of controlled studies." *Frontiers in Psychology* 10 (May 3, 2019): 943.

70   *In areas with more green spaces, the risk of cardiovascular disease is decreased*: Gascon, M., M. Triguero-Mas, D. Martínez, P. Dadvand, D. Rojas-Rueda, A. Plasència, and M.J. Nieuwenhuijsen. "Residential green spaces and mortality: A systematic review." *Environment International* 86 (January 2016): 60–67.

70   *"green exercise" ... results in improvements in mental well-being*: Pretty, J., J. Peacock, M. Sellens, and M. Griffin. "The mental and physical health outcomes of green exercise." *International Journal of Environmental Health Research* 15, no. 5 (2005): 319–37.

70   *"green exercise" ... results in improvements in ... self-esteem*: Peacock, J., R. Hine, and J. Pretty. "Got the blues, then find some greenspace: The mental health benefits of green exercise activities and green care." *Mind Week Report*. Centre for Environment and Society, Department of Biological Sciences, University of Essex (February 2007).

70   *"green exercise" ... results in improvements in ... depression*: Barton, J., R. Hine and J. Pretty. "The health benefits of walking in greenspaces of high natural and heritage value." *Journal of Integrative Environmental Sciences* 6, no. 4 (2009): 261–78.

70   *Being exposed to plants decreases levels of the stress hormone cortisol, resting heart rate, and blood pressure*: Park, B.J., Y. Tsunetsugu, T. Kasetani, T. Kagawa, and Y. Miyazaki. "The physiological effects of Shinrin-yoku (taking in the forest atmosphere or forest bathing): Evidence from field

experiments in 24 forests across Japan." *Environmental Health and Preventive Medicine* 15, no. 1 (January 2010): 18–26.

71   *simply looking at pictures of nature can lower your blood pressure, stress, and mental fatigue*: Hartig, T., M. Mang, and G.W. Evans. "Restorative effects of natural environment experience." *Environment and Behavior* 23 (January 1, 1991): 3–26.

71   *Research has shown that images containing water are more restorative than those without*: White, M.P., A. Smith, K. Humphries, S. Pahl, D. Snelling, and M.H. Depledge. "Blue space: The importance of water for preference, affect and restorative ratings of natural and built scenes." *Journal of Environmental Psychology* 30, no. 4 (December 2010): 482–93.

71   *natural environments decrease stress and mental fatigue by promoting fascination*: Kaplan, S. "The restorative benefits of nature: Toward an integrative framework." *Journal of Psychology* 15 (1995): 169–82.

72   *find 120 minutes per week to spend outside in a natural environment*: White, M.P., I. Alcock, J. Grellier, B.W. Wheeler, T. Hartig, S.L. Warber, A. Bone, M.H. Depledge, and L.E. Fleming. "Spending at least 120 minutes a week in nature is associated with good health and well-being." *Scientific Reports* 9, no. 1 (June 13, 2019): 7730.

72–73   *3 days in natural surroundings restores our brain function and sense of wellness*: Strayer, D.L. "Cognition in the Wild." Invited keynote presentation at the Nature Bridge Evening on the Lake, held in Seattle, WA (March 11, 2016).

73   *the benefits of immersion in a natural setting begin to show after only 5 minutes*: Barton, J., and J. Pretty. "What is the best dose of nature and green exercise for improving mental health? A multi-study analysis." *Journal of Environmental Science and Technology* 44, no. 10 (May 15, 2010): 3947–55.

73   *their results can be used to shape public policy and better environments where people live*: Pretty, J., M. Rogerson, and J. Barton. "Green mind theory: How brain-body-behaviour links into natural and social environments for healthy habits." *International Journal of Environmental Research and Public Health* 14, no. 7 (June 30, 2017): pii E706.

76   *Dr. Drew Ramsey . . . treats anxiety and depression*: Schiffman, R. "Can what we eat affect how we feel?" *New York Times* (March 28, 2019). Available at www.nytimes.com/2019/03/28/well/eat/food-mood-depression-anxiety-nutrition-psychiatry.html.

78   *In an article for* Harvard Health, *Dr. Uma Naidoo makes a case*: Naidoo, U. "Gut feelings: How food affects your mood." *Harvard Health Blog* (December 7, 2018). Available at www.health.harvard.edu/blog/gut-feelings-how-food-affects-your-mood-2018120715548.

STEP 3: PRACTISE RADICAL ATTENTION

83   *They came up with a simple formula for performance that is incredibly powerful*: stress plus rest equals growth: Stulberg, B., and S. Magness. *Peak Performance: Elevate Your Game, Avoid Burnout, and Thrive with the New Science of Success*. New York, NY: Rodale Books, 2017.

85–86   *Later, writing in the* Player's Tribune, *Bautista described*: Bautista, J. "Are you flipping kidding me?" *Player's Tribune* (November 9, 2015). Available at www.theplayerstribune.com/en-us/articles/jose-bautista-bat-flip.

86   *a three-step method to help prevent distractions from taking over your attention*: Moore, M., E. Phillips, and J. Hanc. *Organize Your Mind, Organize Your Life: Train Your Brain to Get More Done in Less Time*. New York, NY: Harlequin, 2011.

87   *by practising certain attitudes and lifestyle choices, and performing mental exercises like playing music*: The Brain Science Behind Business (Harvard Business Review Special Issue) (January 22, 2019): 90.

90   *Words of Wisdom: John Foley*: Episode 1 of *The Dr. Greg Wells Podcast*. "John Foley on Glad to Be Here" (September 4, 2018). Available at https://anchor.fm/dr-greg-wells/episodes/1--John-Foley-on-Glad-To-Be-Here-e1rjmj.

93   *superior frontal lobe of the brain, the inferior parietal lobe, and the superior temporal cortex*: Hopfinger, J.B., M.H. Buonocore, and G.R. Mangun. "The neural mechanisms of top-down attentional control." *Nature Neuroscience* 3, no. 3 (March 2000): 284–91.

93   *The inferior frontal cortex also appears to play a role in attention and inhibition*: Sebastian, A., P. Jung, J. Neuhoff, M. Wibral, P.T. Fox, K. Lieb, P. Fries, S.B. Eickhoff, O. Tüscher, and A. Mobascher. "Dissociable attentional and inhibitory networks of dorsal and ventral areas of the right inferior frontal cortex: A combined task-specific and coordinate-based meta-analytic fMRI study." *Brain Structure and Function* 221, no. 3 (April 2016): 1635–51.

94   *change structures in the brain called the* anterior cingulate cortex: Tang, Y.Y., B.K. Hölzel, and M.I. Posner. "The neuroscience of mindfulness meditation." *Nature Reviews Neuroscience* 16, no. 4 (April 2015): 213–25.

94   *change structures in the brain called . . . the* inferior frontal cortex: Hampshire, A., S.R. Chamberlain, M.M. Monti, J. Duncan, and A.M. Owen. "The role of the right inferior frontal gyrus: Inhibition and attentional control." *Neuroimage* 50, no. 3 (April 15, 2010): 1313–19.

95   *"the awareness that emerges . . . the unfolding of experience moment by moment"*: Kabat-Zinn, J. "Mindfulness-based interventions in context: Past, present, and future." *Clinical Psychology Science and Practice* 10, no. 2 (2003): 144–56.

95   *practising living in the moment and controlling your attention*: Moore, A., T. Gruber, J. Derose, and P. Malinowski. "Regular, brief mindfulness meditation practice improves electrophysiological markers of attentional control." *Frontiers in Human Neuroscience* 6 (February 10, 2012): 18.

96   *unravelling the physiological mechanisms that explain the benefits*: Malinowski, P. "Neural mechanisms of attentional control in mindfulness meditation." *Frontiers in Neuroscience* 7 (February 4, 2013): 8.

96   *8 weeks of mindfulness-based stress-reduction (MSBR) meditation resulted in an increase*: Hölzel, B.K., J. Carmody, M. Vangel, C. Congleton, S.M. Yerramsetti, T. Gard, and S.W. Lazar. "Mindfulness practice leads to increases in regional brain gray matter density." *Psychiatry Research* 191, no. 1 (January 30, 2011): 36–43.

96   *mindfulness meditation improves outcomes for people with anxiety*: Fadel, Z., K.T. Martucci, R.A. Kraft, J.G. McHaffie, and R.C. Coghill. "Neural correlates of mindfulness meditation-related anxiety relief." *Social Cognitive and Affective Neuroscience* 9, no. 6 (June 2014): 751–59.

96   *Mindfulness training has also been shown to be helpful for people struggling with addictions and eating disorders*: Kristeller, J.L., and R.Q. Wolever. "Mindfulness-based eating awareness training for treating binge eating disorder: The conceptual foundation." *Eating Disorders* 19 (January–February 2011): 49–61.

96   *Mindfulness training has also been shown to be helpful for . . . attention deficit hyperactivity disorder*: Zylowska, L., D.L. Ackerman, M.H. Yang, J.L. Futrell, N.L. Horton, T.S. Hale, C. Pataki, and S.L. Smalley. "Mindfulness meditation training in adults and adolescents with ADHD: A feasibility study." *Journal of Attention Disorders* 11, no. 6 (May 2008): 737–46.

96   *Mindfulness training has also been shown to be helpful for . . . recurrent depression*: Kuyken, W., S. Byford, R.S. Taylor, E. Watkins, E. Holden, K. White, B. Barrett, R. Byng, A. Evans, E. Mullan, and J.D. Teasdale. "Mindfulness-based cognitive therapy to prevent relapse in recurrent depression." *Journal of Consulting and Clinical Psychology* 76, no. 6 (December 2008): 966–78.

96   *Mindfulness training has also been shown to be helpful for . . . severe mental illnesses*: Davis, L., and S. Kurzban. "Mindfulness-based treatment for people with severe mental illness: A literature review." *American Journal of Psychiatric Rehabilitation* 15, no. 2 (April 2012): 202–32.

96   *attitudinal qualities of mindfulness training were credited for driving many of the benefits related to increasing resilience*: Chin, B., E.K. Lindsay, C.M. Greco, K.W. Brown, J.M. Smyth, A.G.C. Wright, and J.D. Creswell.

"Psychological mechanisms driving stress resilience in mindfulness training: A randomized controlled trial." *Health Psychology* 38, no. 8 (May 23, 2019): 759–68.

96   *meditation also appears to protect the grey matter in the brain from age-related decline*: Luders, E., N. Cherbuin, and F. Kurth. "Forever young(er): Potential age-defying effects of long-term meditation on gray matter atrophy." *Frontiers in Psychology* 5 (January 21, 2015): 1551.

96–97   *mindfulness is now becoming standard practice for progressive athletes and coaches to enhance human performance*: Bühlmayer, L., D. Birrer, P. Röthlin, O. Faude, and L. Donath. "Effects of mindfulness practice on performance-relevant parameters and performance outcomes in sports: A meta-analytical review." *Sports Medicine* (Auckland, New Zealand) 47, no. 11 (November 2017): 2309–21.

97   *improving their ability to focus and control their attention; reducing anxiety, stress, and burnout*: Li, C., Y. Zhu, M. Zhang, H. Gustafsson, and T. Chen. "Mindfulness and athlete burnout: A systematic review and meta-analysis." *International Journal of Environmental Research and Public Health* 16, no. 3 (February 3, 2019): E449.

97   *enhancing their ability to enter into flow states*: Scott-Hamilton, J., N.S. Schutte, and R.F. Brown. "Effects of a mindfulness intervention on sports-anxiety, pessimism, and flow in competitive cyclists." *Applied Psychology: Health and Well Being* 8, no. 1 (March 2016): 85–103.

97   *an increase in the activation of the "experiential network"*: Garrison, K.A., T.A. Zeffiro, D. Scheinost, R.T. Constable, and J.A. Brewer. "Meditation leads to reduced default mode network activity beyond an active task." *Cognitive, Affective and Behavioral Neuroscience* 15, no. 3 (September 2015): 712–20.

97   *networks in the brain related to the ability to control focus and attention become more active and strengthened*: Malinowski, P. "Neural mechanisms of attentional control in mindfulness meditation." *Frontiers in Neuroscience* 7 (February 4, 2013): 8.

102   *walking before a mental task can help you do that task better*: McMorris, T., and B.J. Hale. "Differential effects of differing intensities of acute exercise on speed and accuracy of cognition: A meta-analytical investigation." *Brain and Cognition* 80, no. 3 (December 2012): 338–51.

102   *improved reaction time on the Stroop Test after the exercise session ended*: Yanagisawa, H., I. Dan, D. Tsuzuki, M. Kato, M. Okamoto, Y. Kyutoku, and H. Soya. "Acute moderate exercise elicits increased dorsolateral prefrontal activation and improves cognitive performance with Stroop Test." *Neuroimage* 50, no. 4 (May 1, 2010): 1702–10.

102   *an increase in cognitive performance matched by improvements in blood flow and oxygenation of the brain*: Endo, K., K. Matsukawa, N. Liang, C. Nakatsuka, H. Tsuchimochi, H. Okamura, and T. Hamaoka. "Dynamic exercise improves cognitive function in association with increased prefrontal oxygenation." *Journal of Physiological Sciences* 63, no. 4 (July 2013): 287–98.

102   *short bouts of exercise . . . improve your mood and make you feel more energetic*: Miller, J.C., and Z. Krizan. "Walking facilitates positive affect (even when expecting the opposite)." *Emotion* (Washington, DC) 16, no. 5 (August 2016): 775–85.

102   *breathing, meditation, and posture-based yoga increased overall brainwave activity*: Desai, R., A. Tailor, and T. Bhatt. "Effects of yoga on brainwaves and structural activation: A review." *Complementary Therapies in Clinical Practice* 21, no. 2 (May 2015): 112–18.

103   *cardiorespiratory endurance—how fit our heart, lungs, blood, and muscles are—has a positive effect on our brain function*: Prakash, R.S., M.W. Voss, K.I. Erickson, J.M. Lewis, L. Chaddock, E. Malkowski, H. Alves, J. Kim, A. Szabo, S.M. White, et al. "Cardiorespiratory fitness and attentional control in the aging brain." *Frontiers in Human Neuroscience* 4 (January 14, 2011): 229.

105   *several effects occur when we expose ourselves to cold*: White, G.E., and G.D. Wells. "Cold-water immersion and other forms of cryotherapy: Physiological changes potentially affecting recovery from high-intensity exercise." *Extreme Physiology and Medicine* 2, no. 1 (September 1, 2013): 26.

105   *athletes who sit in cold tubs after training or games*: Bleakley, C., S. McDonough, E. Gardner, G.D. Baxter, J.T. Hopkins, and G.W. Davison. "Cold-water immersion (cryotherapy) for preventing and treating muscle soreness after exercise." *Cochrane Database of Systematic Reviews* 2, no. CD008262 (February 15, 2012).

105   *cold therapy not only causes our core temperature to reduce, but induces cardiovascular and endocrine changes as well*: White, G.E., and G.D. Wells. "Cold-water immersion and other forms of cryotherapy: Physiological changes potentially affecting recovery from high-intensity exercise." *Extreme Physiology and Medicine* 2, no. 1 (September 1, 2013): 26.

105   *increase the release of noradrenaline in the synapses of the neurons of the brain*: Shevchuk, N.A. "Adapted cold shower as a potential treatment for depression." *Medical Hypotheses* 70, no. 5 (2008): 995–1001.

105   *Beta-endorphins are known to produce feelings of euphoria*: Veening, J.G., and H.P. Barendregt. "The effects of beta-endorphin: State change modification." *Fluids and Barriers of the CNS* 12 (January 29, 2015): 3.

105   *help to diminish activity in areas of the brain related to stress—the same effects produced by running and meditation*: Harte, J.L., G.H. Eifert, and R. Smith. "The effects of running and meditation on beta-endorphin, corticotropin-releasing hormone and cortisol in plasma, and on mood." *Biological Psychology* 40, no. 3 (June 1995): 251–65.

106   *Dr. Geert Buijze conducted a study*: Beard, A. "Cold showers lead to fewer sick days." *Harvard Business Review* (March–April 2018): 34–35.

106   *researchers described a 24-year-old woman with symptoms of major depressive disorder*: van Tulleken, C., M. Tipton, H. Massey, and C.M. Harper. "Open water swimming as a treatment for major depressive disorder." *BMJ Case Reports* (August 21, 2018).

108   *A work environment that is too hot or too cold can impact your attention and focus*: Cornell University. "Study links warm offices to fewer typing errors and higher productivity." *ScienceDaily* (October 22, 2004).

108   *the magic temperature for working on mental tasks is 22°C*: Seppänen, O., W.J. Fisk, and Q.H. Lei. "Effect of temperature on task performance in office environment." Conference proceedings. 5th International Conference on Cold Climate Heating, Ventilating and Air Conditioning. (July 2006): 1–11.

108   *there is a danger that you may blow off your carbon dioxide*: Datta, A., and M. Tipton. "Respiratory responses to cold water immersion: Neural pathways, interactions, and clinical consequences awake and asleep." *Journal of Applied Physiology* (Bethesda, MD: 1985) 100, no. 6 (June 2006): 2057–64.

108   *the "cold-shock" response, which is very dangerous*: Tipton, M.J. "The initial responses to cold-water immersion in man." *Clinical Science* (London, England: 1979) 77, no. 6 (December 1989): 581–88.

109   *The constant distraction leads to higher levels of distress and leaves us feeling burned out and exhausted*: Krabbe, D., S. Ellbin, M. Nilsson, I.H. Jonsdottir, and H. Samuelsson. "Executive function and attention in patients with stress-related exhaustion: Perceived fatigue and effect of distraction." *Stress* (Amsterdam, Netherlands) 20, no. 4 (July 2017): 333–40.

109   *In his book* The Five Thieves of Happiness: Izzo, J.B. *The Five Thieves of Happiness*. San Francisco, CA: Berrett-Koehler Publishers, 2017.

112   *Words of Wisdom: Dr. Brynn Winegard*: Episode 2 of *The Dr. Greg Wells Podcast*. "Brynn Winegard on the Neuroscience of Mental Health and Performance" (September 6, 2018). Available at https://anchor.fm/dr-greg-wells/episodes/2--Dr--Brynn-Winegard-on-the-Neuroscience-of-Mental-Health-and-Performance-e1rjqh.

STEP 4: DO LESS (TO ACHIEVE MORE)

115   *In a creative state, our mind is open, curious, and spontaneous*: Lopata, J.,
E.A. Nowicki, and M.F. Joanisse. "Creativity as a distinct trainable mental state: An EEG study of musical improvisation." *Neuropsychologia* 99 (May 2017): 246–58.

116   *"I am enough of the artist to draw freely . . . Imagination encircles the world"*:
Viereck, G.S. "What life means to Einstein: An interview by George Sylvester Viereck." *Saturday Evening Post* (October 26, 1929): 17.

116   *IBM Global CEO study identified creativity as the most important leadership quality*: Andrew, J.P., J. Manget, D.C. Michael, A. Taylor, and H. Zablit. "Innovation 2010: A return to prominence—and the emergence of a new world order." *BCG Report*. Boston, MA: Boston Consulting Group, April 2010: 1–23.

117   *the role that neural structures in the brain play in the biological roots of creativity*: Shiv, B. "Baba Shiv: How do you find breakthrough ideas?" *Insights by Stanford Business* (October 15, 2013). Available at https://www.gsb .stanford.edu/insights/baba-shiv-how-do-you-find-breakthrough-ideas.

118   *When the climb had just been completed, videographer Jimmy Chin said some interesting things about Honnold*: Chin, J. [No title.] Instagram (June 4, 2017). Available at www.instagram.com/p/BU7HGGaDS9c /?utm_source=ig_embed.

122   *Words of Wisdom: Ariel Garten*: Episode 15 of *The Dr. Greg Wells Podcast*. "Ariel Garten on Building Muse and the Neuroscience of Meditation" (December 11, 2018). Available at https://anchor.fm/dr-greg-wells /episodes/15--Ariel-Garten-on-Building-Muse-and-the-Neuroscience -of-Meditation-e1sv6l.

124   *Athletes use rituals to help themselves calm down*: Harvey-Jenner, C. "These are the clever tricks Olympic athletes use to overcome anxiety." *Cosmopolitan* (UK) (August 19, 2016). Available at https://www.cosmopolitan .com/uk/body/health/news/a45436/breathing-techniques-tricks-calm -anxiety-olympic-athletes/.

125   *deliberately smiling can help decrease levels of the stress hormone cortisol*: Martin, J.D., H.C. Abercrombie, E. Gilboa-Schechtman, and P.M. Niedenthal. "Functionally distinct smiles elicit different physiological responses in an evaluative context." *Scientific Reports* 8, no. 1 (March 1, 2018): 3558.

125   *dopamine, endorphins, and serotonin—are all released when you smile*: Lane, R.D. "Neural correlates of conscious emotional experience." In Lane, R.D., and L. Nadel (eds.). *Series in Affective Science: Cognitive Neuroscience of Emotion*. New York, NY: Oxford University Press, 2000: 354–70.

128   *Words of Wisdom*: *Dr. Ellen Choi*: Episode 6 of *The Dr. Greg Wells Podcast*. "Dr. Ellen Choi on the Art and Science of Mindfulness" (October 9, 2018). Available at https://anchor.fm/dr-greg-wells/episodes/6--Dr--Ellen -Choi-on-the-Art-and-Science-of-Mindfulness-e1rjr9.

130   *People who meditate regularly experience a 23% reduction in all-cause mortality*: Levine, G.N., R.A. Lange, C.N. Bairey-Merz, R.J. Davidson, K. Jamerson, P.K. Mehta, E.D. Michos, K. Norris, I.B. Ray, K.L. Saban, et al. "Meditation and cardiovascular risk reduction: A scientific statement from the American Heart Association." *Journal of the American Heart Association* 6, no. 10 (September 28, 2017): e002218.

131   *regular meditation helps to change the responses of a region of the brain called the* amygdala: Levine, G.N., R.A. Lange, C.N. Bairey-Merz, R.J. Davidson, K. Jamerson, P.K. Mehta, E.D. Michos, K. Norris, I.B. Ray, K.L. Saban, et al. "Meditation and cardiovascular risk reduction: A scientific statement from the American Heart Association." *Journal of the American Heart Association* 6, no. 10 (September 28, 2017): e002218.

131   *meditation improves mood, stress, and hormone levels and can reduce anxiety, pain, and depression*: Taren, A.A., P.J. Gianaros, C.M. Greco, E.K. Lindsay, A. Fairgrieve, K.W. Brown, R.K. Rosen, J.L. Ferris, E. Julson, A.L. Marsland, et al. "Mindfulness meditation training alters stress-related amygdala resting state functional connectivity: A randomized controlled trial." *Social Cognitive and Affective Neuroscience* 10, no. 12 (December 2015): 1758–68.

131   *we create something called* brain-derived neurotrophic factor: Saeed, S.A., K. Cunningham, and R.M. Bloch. "Depression and anxiety disorders: Benefits of exercise, yoga, and meditation." *American Family Physician* 99, no. 10 (May 15, 2019): 620–27.

132   *meditating a few times per week . . . can increase the grey matter in the parts of the brain responsible for emotional regulation and learning*: Cahn, B.R., M.S. Goodman, C.T. Peterson, R. Maturi, and P.J. Mills. "Yoga, meditation and mind–body health: Increased BDNF, cortisol awakening response, and altered inflammatory marker expression after a 3-month yoga and meditation retreat." *Frontiers in Human Neuroscience* 11 (June 26, 2017): 315.

133–34 *Meditation is an effortful training practice that involves learning about the transient nature of thoughts and thought patterns*: Last, N., E. Tufts, and L.E. Auger. "The effects of meditation on grey matter atrophy and neurodegeneration: A systematic review." *Journal of Alzheimer's Disease* 56, no. 1 (2017): 275–86.

134   *MAP training approach can have a significant positive impact on symptoms of various conditions, such as depression*: Shors, T.J., R.L. Olson, M.E.

Bates, E.A. Selby, and B.L. Alderman. "Mental and physical (MAP) training: A neurogenesis-inspired intervention that enhances health in humans." *Neurobiology of Learning and Memory* 115 (November 2014): 3–9; Alderman, B.L., R.L. Olson, C.J. Brush, and T.J. Shors. "MAP training: Combining meditation and aerobic exercise reduces depression and rumination while enhancing synchronized brain activity." *Translational Psychiatry* 6 (February 2, 2016): e726.

134   *it stimulates neurogenesis—the growth of new neurons in the brain*: Shors, T.J., R.L. Olson, M.E. Bates, E.A. Selby, and B.L. Alderman. "Mental and physical (MAP) training: A neurogenesis-inspired intervention that enhances health in humans." *Neurobiology of Learning and Memory* 115 (November 2014): 3–9.

135   *sauna bathing is a powerful practice that has health benefits for your body and brain*: Laukkanen, J.A., T. Laukkanen, and S.K. Kunutsor. "Cardiovascular and other health benefits of sauna bathing: A review of the evidence." *Mayo Clinic Proceedings* 93, no. 8 (August 2018): 1111–21.

135   *people who engaged in frequent sauna use had reduced risks of fatal cardiovascular events*: Laukkanen, T., H. Khan, F. Zaccardi, A. Jari, and J.A. Laukkanen. "Association between sauna bathing and fatal cardiovascular and all-cause mortality events." *JAMA Internal Medicine* 175, no. 4 (April 2015): 542–48.

135   *those who took them two to three times weekly were 12% less likely to have a stroke*: Kunutsor, S.K., H. Khan, F. Zaccardi, T. Laukkanen, P. Willeit, and J.A. Laukkanen. "Sauna bathing reduces the risk of stroke in Finnish men and women." *Neurology* 90, no. 22 (May 2018): e1937–44.

136   *there may be positive health effects for people with inflammatory conditions*: Hussain, J., and M. Cohen. "Clinical effects of regular dry sauna bathing: A systematic review." *Evidence-Based Complementary and Alternative Medicine* (April 24, 2018): 1857413.

136   *blood, arterial stiffness, and cardiovascular system markers were all observed to improve*: Laukkanen, T., K.S. Kunutsor, F. Zaccardi, E. Lee, P. Willeit, H. Khan and J.A. Laukkanen. "Acute effects of sauna bathing on cardiovascular function." *Journal of Human Hypertension* 32 (February 2018): 129–38.

136   *sauna exposure seems to decrease the risk of Alzheimer's disease and dementia*: Laukkanen, T., S. Kunutsor, J. Kauhanen, and J.A. Laukkanen. "Sauna bathing is inversely associated with dementia and Alzheimer's disease in middle-aged Finnish men." *Age and Ageing* 46, no. 2 (March 1, 2017): 245–49.

136   *networks of neurons in the brain are more relaxed and some cognitive processes can be performed more efficiently*: Cernych, M., A. Satas, and M. Brazaitis.

"Post-sauna recovery enhances brain neural network relaxation and improves cognitive economy in oddball tasks." *International Journal of Hyperthermia* 35, no. 1 (2018): 375–82.

136   *Benefits include increased growth hormone levels*: Hannuksela, M.L., and S. Ellahham. "Benefits and risks of sauna bathing." *American Journal of Medicine* 110 (2001): 118–26.

136   *Benefits include . . . muscle regrowth after training*: Selsby, J.T., S. Rother, S. Tsuda, O. Pracash, J. Quindry, and S.L. Dodd. "Intermittent hyperthermia enhances skeletal muscle regrowth and attenuates oxidative damage following reloading." *Journal of Applied Physiology* 102 (1985): 1702–7.

136   *Benefits include . . . increased blood volume*: Costa, R.J.S., M.J. Crockford, J.P. Moore, and N.P. Walsh. "Heat acclimation responses of an ultra-endurance running group preparing for hot desert-based competition." *European Journal of Sport Science* 14, no. 1 (March 19, 2012): S131–41.

136   *Benefits include . . . increased overall endurance*: Sawka, M.N., C.B. Wanger, and K.B. Pandolf. "Thermoregulatory responses to acute exercise-heat stress and heat acclimation." *Handbook of Physiology, Environmental Physiology* (January 1, 2011).

136   *although sauna bathing is safe for most people, there are risks*: Hannuksela, M.L., and S. Ellahham. "Benefits and risks of sauna bathing." *American Journal of Medicine* 110 (2001): 118–26.

143   *it can be a very powerful stress reducer and can decrease symptoms of depression and anxiety*: Jayakody, K., S. Gunadasa, and C. Hosker. "Exercise for anxiety disorders: Systematic review." *British Journal of Sports Medicine* 48, no. 3 (February 2014): 187–96.

145   *Charles Darwin built a path*: Gross, J. "Walking meetings? 5 surprising thinkers who swore by them." *TED Blog* (April 29, 2013). Available at https://blog.ted.com/walking-meetings-5-surprising-thinkers-who-swore-by-them/.

148   *Bob Moritz, the chairman of the professional services firm PwC, was quoted*: Gunaratna, S. "Business leaders urge new thinking in age of artificial intelligence." *CBS News* (January 17, 2017). Available at www.cbsnews.com/news/davos-how-artificial-intelligence-may-change-work-as-we-know-it/.

STEP 5: EMBRACE THE EXTRAORDINARY

155   *Flow was first described by Mihaly Csikszentmihalyi*: Csikszentmihalyi, M. *Flow: The Psychology of Optimal Experience*. New York: Harper & Row, 1990.

156   *"ideal performance state"* . . . *was first described by psychologists Robert M.*
Yerkes and John Dillingham Dodson in 1908: Teigen, K.H. "Yerkes-Dodson:
A law for all seasons." *Theory Psychology* 4 (1994): 525; Privette, G., K.K.
Hwang, and C.M. Bundrick. "Cross-cultural measurement of experience:
Taiwanese and Americans' peak performance, peak experience, misery,
failure, sport, and average events." *Perception and Motor Skills* 84 (3 Pt 2)
(June 1997): 1459–82.

159   *peak experience involves "a heightened sense of wonder, awe, or ecstasy over*
an experience": Privette, G. "Defining moments of self-actualization: Peak
performance and peak experience." In Schneider, K.J., J.F.T. Bugental,
and J.F. Pierson (eds.). *The Handbook of Humanistic Psychology: Leading*
Edges in Theory, Research, and Practice (Chapter 14). Washington, DC:
Sage Publications, 2002.

162   *rhythmic brain responses that have been shown to spike when higher cognitive*
processes are engaged: Rutgers University. "Effect of gamma waves on cognitive and language skills in children." *ScienceDaily* (October 21, 2008).

162   *Gamma waves appear to originate in the base of your brain*: Jia, X., and A.
Kohn. "Gamma rhythms in the brain." *PLOS Biology* 9, no. 4 (April
2011): e1001045.

166   *Phelps went through what many of us experience in our careers and lives: a*
dark period: Scutti, S. "Michael Phelps: 'I am extremely thankful that I did
not take my life.'" *CNN.com* (January 20, 2018). Available at www.cnn
.com/2018/01/19/health/michael-phelps-depression/index.html.

168   *When Ware interviewed people on their deathbeds*: Ware, B. *The Top Five*
Regrets of the Dying. Carlsbad, CA: Hay House Inc., 2012.

170   *people seem to have a high chance of living to become centenarians*:
Buettner, D. "9 lessons from the world's Blue Zones on living a long,
healthy life." World Economic Forum Annual Meeting of the New
Champions (January 26, 2017). Available at https://fr.weforum.org
/events/annual-meeting-of-the-new-champions-2017/sessions/the
-blue-zones-of-happiness.

170   *"The people we surround ourselves with . . . As we say, belong to live long"*:
Buettner, D. "Reverse engineering longevity." *Blue Zones* (November
2016). Available at www.bluezones.com/2016/11/power-9/.

171   *Google studied hundreds of its own teams and discovered this: How a*
team functions is far more important than who is on it: Duhigg, C. "What
Google learned from its quest to build the perfect team." *New York*
Times (February 25, 2016). Available at www.nytimes.com/2016/02/28
/magazine/what-google-learned-from-its-quest-to-build-the-perfect
-team.html.

174   *Words of Wisdom: Alex Hutchinson*: Episode 3 of *The Dr. Greg Wells Podcast*. "Alex Hutchinson on the Limits of Human Performance" (September 11, 2018). Available at https://anchor.fm/dr-greg-wells/episodes/3--Alex-Hutchinson-on-the-Limits-of-Human-Performance-e1rjrg.

175   *Gratitude has even been shown to reduce mental-health disorders such as depression*: Sherman, A.C., S. Simonton-Atchley, C.E. O'Brien, D. Campbell, R.M. Reddy, B. Guinee, L.D. Wagner, and P.J. Anderson. "Longitudinal associations between gratitude and depression 1 year later among adult cystic fibrosis patients." *Journal of Behavioral Medicine* (June 28, 2019).

175   *a "gratitude attitude" reduces stress, lowers heart rate*: Kyeong, S., J. Kim, D.J. Kim, H.E. Kim, and J.J. Kim. "Effects of gratitude meditation on neural network functional connectivity and brain-heart coupling." *Scientific Reports* 7, no. 1 (July 11, 2017): 5058.

175   *a "gratitude attitude" . . . decreases inflammation in the body*: Moieni, M., M.R. Irwin, K.E.B. Haltom, I. Jevtic, M.L. Meyer, E.C. Breen, S.W. Cole, and N.I. Eisenberger. "Exploring the role of gratitude and support-giving on inflammatory outcomes." *Emotion* 19, no. 6 (September 2019): 939–49.

176   *Gratitude generates kind-hearted acts*: Ma, L.K., R.J. Tunney, and E. Ferguson. "Does gratitude enhance prosociality? A meta-analytic review." *Psychological Bulletin* 143, no. 6 (June 2017): 601–35.

177   *Music can help energize your body, activate your brain, reduce fatigue, and increase your performance*: Bacon, C.J., T.R. Myers, and C.I. Karageorghis. "Effect of music-movement synchrony on exercise oxygen consumption." *Journal of Sports Medicine and Physical Fitness* 52, no. 4 (August 2012): 359–65.

177   *if we listen to music while exercising, our bodies pick up on the pace and flow of the music and start to mirror it*: Bernardi, L., C. Porta, and P. Sleight. "Cardiovascular, cerebrovascular, and respiratory changes induced by different types of music in musicians and non-musicians: The importance of silence." *Heart* 92, no. 4 (April 2006): 445–52.

177   *Music can even make a tough workout feel easier to complete*: Karageorghis, C.I., D.A. Mouzourides, D.L. Priest, T.A. Sasso, D.J. Morrish, and C.J. Walley. "Psychophysical and ergogenic effects of synchronous music during treadmill walking." *Journal of Sport and Exercise Psychology* 31, no. 1 (February 2009): 18–36.

177   *music can also have an important effect on your brain's ability to execute*: Schlaug, G. "Musicians and music making as a model for the study of brain plasticity." *Progress in Brain Research* 217 (2015): 37–55.

178   *a literature review that documents the effects of music on individuals and groups*: Koelsch, S. "Brain correlates of music-evoked emotions." *Nature Reviews Neuroscience* 15, no. 3 (March 2014): 170–80.

INDEX

CONNECT AND LEARN MORE

I'm so honoured that you joined me on this journey. I hope this book has been helpful and makes your life better. I look forward to hearing how you are resting, refocusing, and recharging.

- Follow me on Twitter and Instagram @drgregwells

- Connect with me on LinkedIn (linkedin.com/in /drgregwells)

- Find loads of resources, including my blog and books, at drgregwells.com

- Access academic and corporate performance programs at wellsperformance.com

- Download Viivio, my elite health and performance app, at viivio.com

- Access digital training programs based on both this and my previous book *The Ripple Effect* at wellsperformance.com/online-training

- Book me for speaking engagements at drgregwells .com/speaking

- Listen and subscribe to the Dr. Greg Wells Podcast at drgregwells.com/podcast or on Anchor at anchor .fm/dr-greg-wells

Thanks for reading this book.
I look forward to connecting with you!

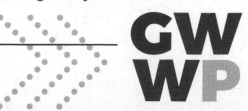